Make the Day Matter!

D1377358

Make the Day Matter!

Promoting Typical Lifestyles
for Adults with Significant Disabilities

by

Pamela M. Walker, Ph.D.
Center on Human Policy
Syracuse University
New York

and

Patricia Rogan, Ph.D.
Indiana University School of Education
Indianapolis

with invited contributors

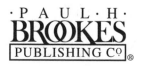
·P A U L·H·
BROOKES
PUBLISHING CO.®

Baltimore • London • Sydney

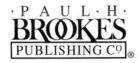

Paul H. Brookes Publishing Co.
Post Office Box 10624
Baltimore, Maryland 21285-0624

www.brookespublishing.com

Typeset by Spearhead Global, Inc., Bear, Delaware.
Manufactured in the United States of America by
Versa Press, Inc., East Peoria, Illinois.

The case studies in this book are composites based on the authors' experiences. In most instances, names and identifying details have been changed to protect confidentiality. In other cases, individual names and stories are used by permission.

The photographs that appear throughout the book are used by permission of the individuals pictured or their parents or guardians.

The views expressed herein are those of the authors and do not necessarily reflect positions of the U.S. government or its agencies.

Library of Congress Cataloging-in-Publication Data

Make the day matter!: Promoting typical lifestyles for adults with significant disabilities /edited by Pamela M. Walker and Patricia Rogan.
    p.   cm.
    Includes index.
    ISBN-13: 978-1-55766-713-7
    ISBN-10: 1-55766-713-6
    1. People with disabilities—Social conditions. 2. People with disabilities—Services for.
    I. Walker, Pamela M. II. Rogan, Patricia, 1956– III. Title.
HV1568.M24 2007
362.4'04—dc22
                                                    2007007704

British Library Cataloguing in Publication data are available from the British Library.

Contents

About the Authors

Pamela M. Walker, Ph.D., Research Project Director, Center on Human Policy, Syracuse University, 805 South Crouse Avenue, Syracuse, NY 13244

Dr. Walker has been a research associate at the Center on Human Policy for the past 25 years. Her research interests include community living, day supports, family supports, recreation/leisure, and social relationships. She has written numerous articles, chapters, and monographs related to these interests.

Patricia Rogan, Ph.D., Professor and Chair of Secondary Education and Area Co-Coordinator of Special Education, Indiana University School of Education, 902 West New York Street, Indianapolis, IN 46202

Dr. Rogan is a professor at the Indiana University School of Education in Indianapolis. She is the current Chair of Secondary Education and Special Education. She prepares school and adult service personnel; provides training and technical assistance at the national, state, and local levels; and conducts research related to transition, employment, and organizational change. Dr. Rogan works closely with Indianapolis schools to develop inclusive education and transition services, as well as with area employment agencies to provide integrated, customized employment services. She is a Small Schools Coach in an urban high school within the Indianapolis Public Schools. Dr. Rogan is a past president of the national APSE: The Network on Employment and has helped coordinate the National Organizational Change conferences and network. She has written numerous articles and book chapters and has co-authored several books, including *Natural Supports in the Workplace: A Manual for Practitioners* (Training Resource Network, 1994) and *Closing the Shop: Conversion from Segregated to Integrated Employment* (Paul H. Brookes Publishing Co., 1994).

About the Contributors

Michael Callahan, President, Marc Gold & Associates, 4101 Gautier-Vancleave Road, Suite 102, Gautier, MS 39553

Mr. Callahan is a native Mississippian and has consulted throughout the United States, Canada, and Europe in the area of employment and transition for the past 25 years. He has worked with Marc Gold & Associates (MG&A) for 27 years and has served as the president of the organization since Marc Gold's untimely death in 1982. MG&A is a network of consultants that provides technical assistance to systems, agencies, and families interested in insuring the complete community participation of persons with severe disabilities. In 2000, Mr. Callahan joined Joe Skiba, Norciva Shumpert, and Melinda Mast to form the nonprofit organization Employment for All (EFA). EFA is dedicated to assuring full access to employment for all persons with disabilities. Mr. Callahan is a co-author of two popular "how-to" books on employment for persons with significant disabilities: *Getting Employed, Staying Employed* (Paul H. Brookes Publishing Co., 1987) and *Keys to the Workplace* (Paul H. Brookes Publishing Co., 1997). He has written numerous articles, chapters, manuals, and curricula pertaining to employment.

Cary Griffin, Senior Partner, Griffin-Hammis Associates, LLC, 5582 Klements Lane, Florence, MT 59833

Mr. Griffin is Senior Partner at Griffin-Hammis Associates, a full-service consultancy specializing in building communities of economic cooperation, creating high-performance organizations, as well as focusing on disability and employment. He is also the co-director of the U.S. Department of Labor's National Self-Employment Technical Assistance, Resources, and Training Project with Virginia Commonwealth University, and former Director of Special Projects at the Rural Institute, University of Montana. Mr. Griffin is also the past director of an adult vocational program in southern Colorado, the former assistant director of the Rocky Mountain Resource and Training Institute, and serves as Founder and former Executive Director of CTAT in Colorado.

Teresa Grossi, Ph.D., Director, Center on Community Living and Careers, Indiana Institute on Disability and Community, Indiana University Center for Excellence, Indiana University, 2853 East Tenth Street, Bloomington, IN 47408

Dr. Grossi is the director for the Center on Community Living and Careers at the Indiana Institute on Disability and Community, the University Center for

Excellence at Indiana University. Dr. Grossi has extensive background in education and employment for individuals with disabilities. She has worked in North Carolina and Ohio as a community-based instructor, transition coordinator, and job coach, and has managed a vocational training program and a supported employment agency. Dr. Grossi serves on a number of editorial boards and has conducted research and written on secondary transition services, community supports, and employment issues for individuals with disabilities. Dr. Grossi serves as President of the National Board for the APSE: The Network on Employment, as a member of the advisory board for the National Postsecondary Outcomes Center, as a member of a research committee for the Division of Career Development and Transition, and as the external evaluator for the National Secondary Transition and Technical Assistance Center.

David Hammis, Senior Partner, Griffin-Hammis Associates, LLC, 317 Franklin Street, Middletown, OH 45042

Mr. Hammis is Senior Partner at Griffin-Hammis Associates, a full-service consultancy specializing in building communities of economic cooperation, creating high-performance organizations, and focusing on disability and employment. He maintains an ongoing relationship with the Rural Institute at the University of Montana, where he served as Project Director for multiple self-employment, employment, and Social Security outreach training and technical assistance projects, including the Rural Institute's Rural Entrepreneurship and Self-Employment Expansion Design Project. Mr. Hammis works with organizations nationally and internationally on self-employment, benefits analysis, supported employment, and employment engineering. He has worked in supported and self-employment since 1988 and is personally responsible for the implementation of thousands of Plans to Achieve Self-Support leading to employment, self-employment, and enhanced personal resources for people with disabilities. In July 1996, Mr. Hammis received the International Association for Persons in Supported Employment Professional of the Year Award for his "outstanding support and commitment to people with disabilities especially in the areas of career development and the use of Social Security Work Incentives."

Jane Harlan-Simmons, M.A., Research Associate, Indiana Institute on Disability and Community at Indiana University, 2853 East Tenth Street, Bloomington, IN 47408

Ms. Harlan-Simmons has been a research associate at the Indiana Institute on Disability and Community (Indiana's University Center for Excellence in Developmental Disabilities) for over 17 years. At the Institute's Center on Aging and Community, Ms. Harlan-Simmons has conducted research, developed model programs, and produced training materials in the fields of aging, disability, and the arts. She has authored journal articles, book chapters, and reports, and has produced videos, media presentations, exhibits, and web pages on topics including community membership, home modification, careers in the arts, and self-expression through creative visual art activities. She has made presentations at conferences and workshops at the national, state, and local levels and provided consultation and technical assistance to a variety of Indiana organizations. Ms. Harlan-Simmons has a master's degree from New York University in Art Therapy.

Richard Luecking, Ed.D., President, TransCen, Inc., 451 Hungerford Drive, Suite 700, Rockville, MD 20850

Dr. Luecking is President of TransCen, Inc., a nonprofit organization based in Rockville, Maryland that is dedicated to improving education and employment outcomes for individuals with disabilities. Dr. Luecking and his TransCen colleagues have been responsible for the design and implementation of numerous model demonstration and research projects related to school-to-work transition and employment of individuals with disabilities. He is the author of a variety of publications on these topics, including his latest book, co-authored by Ellen Fabian and George Tilson, titled *Working Relationships: Creating Career Opportunities for Job Seekers with Disabilities Through Employer Partnerships* (Paul H. Brookes Publishing Co., 2004).

David M. Mank, Ph.D., Director, Indiana Institute on Disability and Community at Indiana University, 2853 East Tenth Street, Bloomington, IN 47408

Dr. Mank is Director of the Indiana Institute on Disability and Community at Indiana University, Indiana's University Center for Excellence on Disabilities. In addition, he is a full professor in the School of Education, Department of Curriculum and Instruction. As a writer and researcher, Dr. Mank has an extensive background in the education and employment for persons with disabilities. He has authored or co-authored more than 100 articles or book chapters. His interests also include a focus on the transition of persons with disabilities from school to adult life and community living. Since 1985, Dr. Mank has maintained responsibility for grant writing and management of more than 40 state or federally funded projects in which he has been Principal Investigator, Director, or Co-director. Dr. Mank holds a bachelor's degree in Psychology and English from Rockhurst College in Kansas City (1975), a master's degree from Portland State University in special education (1977), and a doctorate in special education and rehabilitation from the University of Oregon, Eugene (1985).

Bonnie Shoultz, M.A., Buddhist Chaplain, Center on Human Policy, Syracuse University, 805 South Crouse Avenue, Syracuse, NY 13244

Bonnie Shoultz became a Zen Buddhist nun in 2003. She retired from her position as Associate Director of the Center on Human Policy in 2005 but still does some work at the Center. She is now the Buddhist chaplain at Syracuse University's Hendricks Chapel, as well as a contract chaplain working in correctional/detention settings in Onondaga County under the auspices of Interfaith Works. She has had a long association with the self-advocacy movement in the United States and has worked in the developmental disabilities field since 1974.

Valerie Smith, Ph.D., Assistant Professor, Special Education, Plymouth State University, 17 High Street, Plymouth, NH, 03264

Dr. Smith received her Ph.D. in special education from Syracuse University and is currently an assistant professor of special education at Plymouth State University in New Hampshire. Her research interests are postsecondary education and students with developmental disabilities and partnerships between academic institutions and community organizations.

Jeffrey L. Strully, M.S., Executive Director, Jay Nolan Community Services, 15501 San Fernando Mission Boulevard, Suite # 200, Mission Hills, CA 91390

Mr. Strully is Executive Director of Jay Nolan Community Services. He has held this position for the past 14 years. He has been involved with people with developmental disabilities for over 38 years in a variety of different positions and capacities. In addition, he and his wife are parents of adult children who require long-term support and assistance to live valued lives.

Jennie Todd, B.A., Research Associate, Center on Aging and Community, Indiana Institute on Disability and Community at Indiana University, 2853 East Tenth Street, Bloomington, IN 47408

Ms. Todd has been working and advocating for people with disabilities for over 25 years. She has spent many years developing and implementing some of Indiana's earliest community-based services and developing an agency conversion strategy for closing down her agency's sheltered workshop while facilitating action plans focusing on typical community roles and activities. Currently a research associate at the Center on Aging and Community, Indiana Institute on Disability and Community (Indiana's University Center for Excellence in Developmental Disabilities), Ms. Todd has developed best practice projects and has produced training materials and curricula in the fields of disability, aging, and leadership. She has authored journal articles, book chapters, and has produced videos and media presentations on topics including community membership, person-centered planning, self-determination, and meaningful lives. Ms. Todd has made national, state, and local presentations and provides technical assistance to a variety of state and local organizations.

Perry Whittico, Field Assistant, Grass Roots Organizing Program, Self-Advocacy Association of New York State, Inc., 800 Wilbur Avenue, Suite 3A1, Syracuse, NY 13204

Mr. Whittico has been involved in self-advocacy at the local, state, and national levels for many years. He is a past president and member of Self-Advocates of Central New York and has served as a board member for both the Self-Advocacy Association of New York State, Inc. and Self Advocates Becoming Empowered. He has given many presentations and conducted numerous workshops, locally and nationally, on the topics of self-advocacy, self-determination, and inclusion of people with disabilities on boards and committees. Mr. Whittico is currently a field assistant with the Grass Roots Organizing Program of the Self-Advocacy Association of New York State, Inc.

Foreword

We humans have a breathtaking capacity to invent when we choose to step into the tension between our vision of a desirable future and our current reality. This book invites those responsible for services to people with significant disabilities—advocates, service providers, and policy makers—to stretch our strengths between a vision of days that matter and the current reality of a system that is largely stuck in second best.

The vision is clear. Supporting people with substantial disabilities in real jobs, with career prospects, at good places to work, centers the intentions of the authors of these chapters. Improving children and young people's prospects of taking up such jobs is a central focus of an inclusive and intensely relevant education and the measure of value for the transition activities required by law and rule. Delivering on the job and career interests revealed by thoughtful and daring person-centered plans is the core mission of the work support system and adult services. When people have the dignity of the role of worker in a job that suits them and allows them to contribute, the quest for other socially valued roles as active citizen, association member, householder, and friend becomes somewhat easier and life has a better chance of being good. Those who have been workers have something to retire from rather than being shunted from activity center to senior center.

Those who embrace this vision wholeheartedly know how much creativity it demands. As this book shows, even organizations that employ people with remarkable gifts as self-advocates have more to learn about ensuring good support for great performance. Even dedicated supported employment practitioners have reached only a minority of people who require highly customized employment, so we are nowhere near knowing what the limits of our ability to match people to work may be. Many competitively employed people with substantial disabilities are a long way from having good career prospects and income that lifts them out of poverty. Far too many people are hemmed in to reduced workweeks to protect benefits. Many employed people remain more socially isolated and disengaged than they wish, both at work and outside of work, and some people who have grown up included and gone to work included now wonder if there is a trade-off between inclusion and the intimacy of marriage.

These issues, knotty and sometimes painful as they may be, are a challenge but need not be a worry. For those who are committed to the search for valued social roles as the way to days that matter, this book helps to frame the issues, indicates where and how people are making progress, and underwrites confidence that continued investment in learning will sustain the journey toward equal opportunity regardless of impairment.

The worry is the number of people in the field who have declined the search. Those special educators, rehabilitation counselors, service providers, and system managers who expect people with significant disabilities and their families to celebrate exclusion and be satisfied with a limited range of work that, at best, could only be maintained by underbidding offshore employers or finding a niche for groups of cleaners or yard care workers. And, as this book proves in its first and last chapters, this is not the rump of laggard adopters of supported employment. It is the larger part of the body of expenditure and provision, and it is growing, not shrinking.

Given the evidence amassed in this book and its many references, and given how very many of these references are 10 or more years old, it is hard to work out what confirms people in their limiting beliefs and practices. It is not simple avoidance of supported employment: Many organizations bolt a supported employment service onto their organization chart right next to the sheltered workshop and many newsletters report with pride on the achievements of supported employees right next to the call for more deposits to the activity center's recycling bin. It is not a lack of mandates: This book enumerates the numerous laws and regulations that call for access to customized employment for people with substantial disabilities. It may be a belief that those with substantial disabilities must progress through a continuum of service settings, though lately I hear much less about continua than about maintaining a range of settings in order to allow consumers a choice that suits them or their families (Taylor, 2001). It may be an assumption that work is an all or nothing proposition and that having a job means having no assistance to fill any other social role. It may be lack of external incentives, though given the commitment to deep change demonstrated by the organizations whose accomplishments provide the inspiring content for this book, I am unsure whether extrinsic motivation will turn the trick. It may be a lack of self-efficacy, a belief that people with substantial disabilities have needs so intractably complex or face communities so imperviously rejecting that nothing can be done.

This book will help its readers to rethink their assumptions, inform their practice, and deepen their appreciation about what is possible and what learning lies ahead. But it will take more than that to get unstuck. To encourage substantially more people to step into the tension between a vision of days that matter and our current reality, we need to renew the spirit that made a place for supported employment where there was no place. The messages in this book will not deliver themselves; we need to remember that things began to move more than 25 years ago when committed people brought their convictions to skeptical and sometimes even hostile audiences. The times have changed in important ways, but the necessary qualities of leadership have not. As much as ever, we need to encourage these seven qualities.

1. Impossibly high expectations for what we can learn in order to assist people with substantial disabilities to achieve

2. Close personal partnership with people with substantial disabilities

3. Priority on creating a pathway to success for the people with the least access to opportunity

4. Relentless belief in people's capacity: the limits of current performance outline the shape of what we need to learn in order to be good assistants

5. Opportunism: seizing any opportunity to actually demonstrate what people with substantial disabilities can do

6. Fanatic commitment to show and tell and passion to debate the merits of different approaches

7. Willingness to abandon ineffective or outmoded practices and structures, even when you invented them yourself

This book will help.

John O'Brien
Responsive Systems Associates
58 Willowick Drive
Lithonia, GA 30038

REFERENCE

Taylor, S.J. (2001, February). On choice. *TASH Connections, 27*(2), 8–10.

Note to the Reader

The impetus for this book stemmed from long-term interactions with a variety of stakeholders, including people with disabilities, family members, policy makers, state agency personnel, day and residential service providers, school personnel, and advocates. The book grew out of extensive work to investigate, promote, develop, monitor, and evaluate innovative services and supports for people with significant disabilities. It is an attempt to describe many of the innovations that have affected changes at the federal, state, and local levels, and have resulted in quality outcomes for people with high support needs.

Acknowledgments

There are many people who contributed in one way or another to the completion of this book. We would like to thank all of our co-authors for their important contributions to this book. We are very appreciative of the editorial staff at Brookes, in particular, Rebecca Lazo and Steve Peterson, for their encouragement, patience, and insightful assistance over the long haul in pulling this together. We are also extremely grateful for the ongoing support of our work by family, friends, and colleagues at the Center on Human Policy.

Preparation of this book was supported through a subcontract with the Research and Training Center on Community Living, University of Minnesota, supported by the U.S. Department of Education, Office of Special Education and Rehabilitative Services, National Institute on Disability and Rehabilitation Research (NIDRR), through Contract No. H133B031116.

Make the Day Matter!

Toward Meaningful Daytimes for Adults with Significant Disabilities

PATRICIA ROGAN AND PAMELA M. WALKER

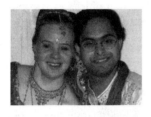

Achieving a meaningful day seems like a simple enough quest. Most adults in our society achieve meaning in their lives in many ways, including engaging in satisfying paid employment, contributing to society through volunteer and other efforts, forming friendships and relationships, learning new things, growing personally and professionally, and engaging in leisure and spiritual endeavors. Unfortunately, adults with disabilities, and especially those with high support needs, continue to struggle to achieve meaningful daytimes. Approximately three out of four (76%) adults with intellectual or developmental disabilities still spend their days in sheltered workshops or segregated day habilitation facilities (Braddock et al., 2005) earning little or no money and having few real choices available to them. Others are grouped in community-based programs largely segregated with others with disabilities, at home with little to do, or working for a limited number of hours each week earning minimal pay, and with little to do when they are not at work (Murphy, Rogan, Handley, Kincaid, & Royce-Davis, 2002).

This dire situation exists today despite the fact that we know better. We know how to support people with disabilities to live full and meaningful lives in the community. There are wonderful examples of innovative practices and quality of life outcomes throughout the United States, Canada, and other countries. Unfortunately, the opportunity to achieve meaningful daytimes is still the exception instead of the rule for adults with disabilities.

LOOKING BACK

It is imperative to know the history of special education and rehabilitation in order to understand what has worked, to better plan for the future, and to avoid the mistakes of the past. The current system of services for youths and adults with significant disabilities has been slow to change. From a history of institutionalization, human services for people with disabilities evolved into an entrenched system of segregated schools, sheltered workshops, segregated day activity centers, mini institutions (e.g., intermediate care facilities), group homes, and separate recreation/leisure options. This separate system has run parallel to regular educational services, typical housing and employment, public transportation, and integrated community and leisure involvement. It has served to keep people with and without disabilities apart, except for those who were paid to provide services to people with disabilities. As a result, this history is replete with stereotypes, misperceptions, stigma, lack of access, and low expectations associated with people with disabilities (Taylor, 1988).

People with disabilities have had to fit into professionally controlled programs such as institutions, sheltered workshops, and group homes if they wanted services because funding has been tied to these facilities. Over time, a continuum of services developed based on a readiness mentality that required people to earn their way into the community by moving from the most restrictive to the least restrictive end of the continuum (Taylor, 1988). The reality, however, was that by spending time in segregated communities, few people were ever considered ready for the community. The following section traces the history of services for people with developmental disabilities (Minnesota Governor's Council on Developmental Disabilities, 2006).

The Era of Institutionalization—1800–1960

The first institutions in the United States opened about 1850 as training schools intended to educate individuals with disabilities. Training schools soon became asylums or custodial institutions that increased in size and in dehumanization (Vail & Thomas, 1966). Overcrowding, understaffing, and segregation led to abuse and neglect. By 1905, there were an average of 500 people per institution and overcrowding worsened. Institutions continued to grow during the 1900s to 200,000 people by 1967, in part due to the inability of families to financially meet the needs of their children with disabilities (especially during the Great Depression), and the lack of educational and other public services.

By the late 19th century, the "incurability" of people with disabilities came to be viewed by medical and charity professionals as a dangerous deviance. The Eugenics Movement arose during this time, as described below.

The Eugenics Movement—1850s–1950s

As the U.S. economy changed from rural to industrial and immigration increased, society's perceptions of people with disabilities changed. There was a growing prejudice toward racial minorities and people with disabilities. "Feeblemindedness" was thought to be hereditary and the root cause of many social problems. The view of people with disabilities as a menace and danger to society peaked around 1920. Such attitudes spurred the rise in eugenics, or the science of the improvement of the human race by better breeding. Proponents of eugenics, many of whom were doctors, advocated for forced sterilization of people with disabilities.

In 1942, the *American Journal of Psychiatry* published a debate on the ethics of killing children with severe disabilities. Foster Kennedy wrote the following, which was endorsed in an unsigned editorial in that publication.

> I believe when the defective child shall have reached the age of 5 years—and on the application of his guardians—that the case should be considered under law by a competent medical board; then it should be reviewed twice more at 4 month intervals; if the board, acting, I repeat, on the applications of the guardians of the child, and after three more examinations of a defective who has reached the age of 5 or more, should decide that the defective has no future hope of one; then I believe it is a merciful and kindly thing to relieve that defective—often tortured and convulsed, grotesque and absurd, useless and foolish, and entirely undesirable—of the agony of living.

It is probable that Hitler's concentration camps and his devotion to eugenics drove the eugenics movement in the United States underground. However, the role of the medical profession continued, as described next.

The Medical Model—1900s

Institutions grew increasingly medical in their orientation. For example, superintendents of institutions were often physicians, institutions were called state hospitals, staff wore white jackets, patients lived on wards, and therapy and treatment were provided. As the president of the American Association on Mental Deficiency stated in 1954, "Medicine, not education, will find the answers" (Minnesota Governor's Planning Council, 2006). The medical model viewed disability as a deficiency or abnormality that resides in the individual. As such, the person with a disability was perceived as deficient and needing to be cured or fixed by a professional. Fortunately, parents began to advocate for more and better services, as described next.

The Parents' Movement—1950–1980

Frustrated by the lack of community services, parents began to organize in the early 1950s. They formed parent groups, including the National Association for Retarded Children (now known as The Arc of the United States), United Cerebral Palsy Association, and Muscular Dystrophy Association. Parents offered educational, social, and other services in such places as their own homes and churches.

Public attitudes slowly began to change as mental retardation "came out of the closet." President John F. Kennedy, whose sister Rosemary had a cognitive disability, launched the President's Panel on Mental Retardation in 1961. Famous people such as Pearl Buck and Dale Evans wrote books about their daughters with disabilities; however, others viewed the books as reinforcing the notion of people with disabilities as "eternal children." An international parent movement was in place by the end of the 1950s.

By the 1960s–1970s, a strong national movement developed, with parents working to challenge conventional wisdom, improve conditions in state institutions, create community services, education and employment opportunities, and initiate legislation and lawsuits. By now, parents were informing professionals and speaking on behalf of their children. The parents' movement today encourages self-advocacy and self-determination of individuals with disabilities. Concurrent with the parent's movement, the concept of normalization was taking root worldwide.

The Principle of Normalization

In 1959, Niels Erik Bank Mikkelsen worked with a group of parents in Denmark on a petition to the government for better treatment of their sons and daughters with disabilities. In this document, they coined the concept of *normalization*, meaning to live according to normal patterns— "making available to [people who are] mentally retarded the patterns and conditions of everyday life which are as close as possible to the norms and patterns of the mainstream of society" (Nirje, 1970). Dr. Bengt Nirje, Secretary General of the Swedish Parent's Association for Mentally Retarded Children, worked to formalize the normalization principle (Nirje, 1970) as follows:

- A normal rhythm of the day (e.g., eating, sleeping)
- A normal routine (e.g., work, school)
- A normal rhythm of the year (e.g., holidays)
- Normal developmental experiences
- The chance to make choices
- The right to live heterosexually (not segregated into "men only" or "women only" accommodations)
- A normal economic standard
- The right to live, work, and play in normal conditions

Denmark and Sweden put the normalization principle into law and Nirje translated the concept to English and published it in the 1969 President's Report on Mental Retardation, which had a significant impact in the United States. Wolf Wolfensberger expanded the concept of normalization and wrote about social role valorization (SRV) (Wolfensberger, 1972), a concept intended to create or support socially valued roles for people in their society. Normalization and SRV spawned a significant human service reform movement in many countries in the last quarter century. The philosophies and practices associated with normalization and SRV offer a clear direction for the field—that services should use socially valued means to promote socially valued lives (O'Brien, 1999). These principles allowed educational integration, supported employment, and community participation to take root and spurred deinstitutionalization (Flynn & Lemay, 1999).

Deinstitutionalization—Mid-1970s–Present

Exposés of the horrible conditions in institutions began as early as 1948 with Albert Deutsch's *The Shame of the State*. In 1965, Senator Robert Kennedy toured Willowbrook State School in New York and spoke of its dehumanizing conditions, calling it a "snakepit" and declaring that Willowbrook State School was not fit for even animals to live in. Burton Blatt and Fred Kaplan followed with their exposé *Christmas in Purgatory* (1974). In 1972, ABC News reporter Geraldo Rivera gained entry to Willowbrook using a stolen key and documented the brutal and horrific living conditions of its residents. The report led to an immediate government inquiry. These exposures served to prompt advocates to sue state governments on the grounds that the confinement and mistreatment of individuals with disabilities was unconstitutional. These lawsuits and public pressure forced professionals and government officials to take action. Initially, efforts to fix institutions were undertaken, but this soon led to changing them to places of last resort, and finally to closing them. When the Education of the Handicapped Act (PL 91-230) was passed in 1970, deinstitutionalization escalated as parents brought their children home to attend local schools.

Despite decades of proof that people with disabilities have a better quality of life in the community, not everyone supports institutional closure. Groups such as the Voice of the Retarded (comprising mostly older parents) support keeping institutions open. In 2005, more than 100,000 people with intellectual and developmental disabilities remained in institutions in the United States (Prouty & Lakin, 2005). The struggle for community living and regular lives continues.

The Independent Living Movement—1970s–Present

Pioneers like Ed Roberts, who is widely acknowledged as the father of the independent living movement, exemplified the core tenets of this movement. Independent living is premised on self-determination about the direction of one's life, making choices, and abiding by those choices. Roberts established the first independent living center (ILC) in Berkeley, California. The Rehabilitation Act of 1993 established ILCs nationally, describing "consumer control of the center regarding decision making, service delivery, management, and establishment of the policy and direction of the center" (Rehabilitation Act of 1993, PL 103-73, Section 725). The 1970s to the present time also saw the development of special education for youth with disabilities.

Special Education

Up until the early 1970s, no state served all children with disabilities. Children were refused services or provided inappropriate programs (Martin, Martin, & Termin, 1996). In response, parents pursued state laws that required local school districts to offer special education to children with disabilities.

The 1971 Pennsylvania Association for Retarded Citizens lawsuit against the Commonwealth of Pennsylvania addressed the exclusion of students with disabilities from school. The landmark decision by a federal district court affirmed the right of youth with disabilities to a free appropriate public education and due process safeguards. It was a predecessor to other litigation. Parent advocacy soon led to the self-advocacy movement.

The Self-Advocacy Movement—1980s–Present

Inspired by the civil rights movement, people with disabilities formed the first self-advocacy group in the United States in 1974 called People First. By 1995 there were over 600 self-advocacy groups in the United States, including the national organization Self Advocates Becoming Empowered, formed in 1991.

In contrast to the medical model, a social model evolved from disability advocates that views disability as a natural part of the human existence. From this perspective, disability is seen as a difference that may derive from the interaction between the individual and society. In other words, disablement is created by oppressive social systems. This theory suggests that the reason some people have a disadvantage is due to a complex form of institutional discrimination. Prejudicial attitudes are learned. The remedy for disability-related problems is to change the nature of interactions between the individual, society members, and the community at large. For example, buildings and transportation can be made accessible through the use of ramps and lifts, poverty and unemployment can be reduced through employment, and negative attitudes and expectations can be changed through education and positive personal experiences with people with disabilities.

Over the years, many people in the disabilities field have learned that segregation begets segregation, that people do not have to get ready for community life in congregate facilities, and that people can live full lives in the community if provided appropriate supports. The barriers to full community participation are seen as stemming from professional and society problems, not from problems in the individual (Bradley, Ashbaugh, & Blaney, 1994). Tables 1.1, 1.2, and 1.3 illustrate some of the contrasting eras of service design over the years.

MAJOR DISABILITY LEGISLATION ·

Between 1968 and 2005, approximately 70 pieces of legislation related to people with disabilities were passed or reauthorized in the United States. This vast and progressive array of legislation has set the tone and direction for disability policy and practices at the state and local levels, including equal rights, access, and appropriate services for youth and adults with disabilities. For example, key legislation has promoted:

• Vocational education and school-to-work transition funds and services for youth with disabilities (e.g., the Vocational Education Act of 1963 [PL 88-210], the School-to-Work Opportunities Act of 1994 [PL 103-239], the

Table 1.1. Focal questions of the era of institutional services

Focal questions	Answers
Who is the person of concern?	The patient
What is the typical setting?	An institution
How are the services organized?	In facilities
What is the model?	Custodial/medical
What are the services?	Care
How are services planned?	Through a plan of care
Who controls the planning decision?	A professional (usually a doctor)
What is the planning context?	Standards of professional practice
What has the highest priority?	Basic needs
What is the objective?	Control or cure

Adapted from Knoll, J. (1992). From community-based alternatives to inclusive communities. *Inclusive Communities, 1*(1), 9.

Carl D. Perkins Vocational Education and Applied Technology Amendments of 1990 [PL 101-392])

- A free appropriate public education for all children with disabilities, including an early intervention system, preschool programs, and support services for transition and assistive technology (e.g., the Education of All Handicapped Children Act of 1975 [PL 94-142] and the Individuals with Disabilities Education Act [IDEA] of 1990 [PL 101-476] Amendments of the Individuals with Disabilities Education Improvement Act of 1991 [PL 102-119] and 1997 [PL 105-17], and 2004 [PL 108-446])

- A program that authorizes cash benefits for people who are blind, disabled, or aged, including special cash payments (Section 1619a) and continued Medicaid eligibility (Section 1619b) for individuals who receive Supplemental Security Income benefits and engage in substantial gainful activity (e.g., the Social Security Act Amendments of 1967 [PL 90-48] and 1983 [PL 98-21])

Table 1.2. Focal questions of the era of deinstitutionalization

Focal questions	Answers
Who is the person of concern?	The client
What is the typical setting?	A group home, workshop, special school, or classroom
How are the services organized?	In a continuum of options
What is the model?	Developmental/behavioral
What are the services?	Programs
How are the services planned?	Through an individualized habilitation plan
Who controls the planning decision?	An interdisciplinary team
What is the planning context?	Team consensus
What had the highest priority?	Skill development, behavior management
What is the objective?	To change behavior

Table 1.3. Focal questions of the era of community membership

Focal questions	Answers
Who is the person of concern?	The citizen
What is the typical setting?	A person's home, local business, the neighborhood school
How are the services organized?	Through a unique array of supports tailored to the individual
What is the model?	Individual support
What are the services?	Supports
How are the services planning?	Through a personal futures plan
Who controls the planning decision?	The individual
What is the planning context?	A circle of support
What has the highest priority?	Self-determination and relationships
What is the objective?	To change the environment and attitudes

- State funding for vocational rehabilitation to provide employment-related services for people with disabilities, including supported employment and transition from school to work, increased access for those with the most significant disabilities, greater consumer choice and control in the rehabilitation process, and opportunities for career advancement (e.g., the Rehabilitation Act of 1973 [PL 93-112] and Amendments of 1986 [PL 99-506] and 1992 [PL 102-569])

- Antidiscrimination against otherwise qualified people with disabilities in any program or activity receiving federal funds (Section 504 of the Rehabilitation Act)

- Low-income rent subsidies to include families consisting of single persons with disabilities (Section 8 of the Housing and Community Development Amendments of 1974 [PL 93-383])

- A bill of rights for persons with developmental disabilities and a system of Protection and Advocacy organizations, Developmental Disabilities Councils, and University Centers on Excellence in each state (e.g., the Developmental Disabilities Assistance and Bill of Rights Act of 1975 [PL 94-103])

- ILCs (e.g., the Rehabilitation, Comprehensive Services, and Developmental Disabilities Amendments of 1978 [PL 95-602])

- Consumer-driven, statewide service delivery systems that increase access to assistive technology devices and services and emphasize advocacy and systems change activities (e.g., the Technology-Related Assistance for Individuals with Disabilities Act of 1988 [PL 100-407] and Amendments of 1994 [PL 103-218])

- Antidiscrimination in housing for people with disabilities (e.g., the Fair Housing Act Amendments of 1988 [PL 100-430])

- The civil rights of people with disabilities by promoting access and prohibiting discrimination in the areas of employment, public services, transportation, public accommodations, and telecommunications (e.g., the Architectural Barriers Act of 1968 [PL 90-480], the Telecommunications for the Disabled Act of 1982 [PL 97-410] and 1996 [PL 104-104], and the Americans with Disabilities Act [ADA] of 1990 [PL 101-336])

- Community supported living arrangements and individualized supports rather than the standardized services common to the intermediate care facilities program (e.g., the Omnibus Budget Reconciliation Act of 1990 [PL 101-508])

The Olmstead Decision

In 1999, the Supreme Court upheld the ADA integration mandate in the case of *Olmstead v. L.C. and E.W.* In rejecting the state of Georgia's appeal to enforce institutionalization of individuals with disabilities, the Supreme Court affirmed the right of individuals with disabilities to live in the "most integrated setting." As a result, the federal government has encouraged states to plan for reforms not only in the health arena but also in the areas of transportation, housing, education, and other social supports to fully integrate people with disabilities into the least restrictive settings. State Olmstead plans have been developed that focus on

- Helping people make the transition from institutions into the community

- Promoting affordable and accessible housing

- Improving the recruitment and retention of direct care workers

- Providing information and referral as well as family-centered assessments

- Allowing funding to follow the individual rather than the providers

- Reducing the waiting lists for home and community-based services

- Increasing employment opportunities for people with disabilities

- Enhancing data collection activities and systems

- Improving transportation that complies with the ADA requirements

However, decreasing revenues and rising Medicaid costs have impeded states' progress toward their Olmstead plan goals (Fox-Grage, Folkemer, & Lewis, 2006). As of 2006, 30 states had developed Olmstead plans (Kitchener, Willmott, Wong, & Harrington, 2006).

The movement toward community integration, self-determination, and individualized supports has required significant shifts in professional and community attitudes, expectations, and behaviors. Professionals are increasingly being pushed to relinquish control of decision making regarding other people's lives, especially as self-advocates have increasingly stepped up and spoken out for choice and control in their own lives. Self-determination and choice initiatives have assisted professionals to see how people with disabilities can control funding and personal support services through the use of individualized budgets (Bradley et al., 2001).

We now find ourselves in an interesting and perplexing situation in the evolution of the disabilities field. On one hand, there are many innovative initiatives and opportunities that have resulted in meaningful daytimes for adults with significant disabilities (e.g., personal budgets, self-employment, homeownership). People with significant disabilities are more visible and involved in our communities than ever before, with greater access to all aspects of our communities. More and more people with disabilities are speaking for themselves and the concepts of self-determination, empowerment, and self-advocacy have widespread support in the community (Lakin & Turnbull, 2005). Media images of people with disabilities have become more positive and public attitudes toward differences have improved.

On the other hand, the exclusion of people with significant disabilities persists in all aspects of life and levels of the system: public schools, residential facilities, sheltered workshops and day activity centers, recreation programs, and elsewhere. Practices of exclusion continue to be justified and "cloaked in whatever rationales make sense for the times" (Jackson, 2006). True systems change has yet to occur in most states and localities. That is, the disability service delivery system continues to be entrenched in outdated models of practice.

CONCEPTUAL FRAMEWORK

This book provides an analysis of our current status in relation to the above paradigm shift, examples of positive practices, challenges we still face, and suggestions for future directions. What is meaningful varies from person to person, depending on one's interests, experiences, and goals. However, all of our lives seem connected by certain elements that are universal and valued. John and Connie Lyle O'Brien's *A Framework for Accomplishment* (1990) provides a wonderful framework for our discussion of meaningful daytimes. Each of the five accomplishments is briefly described:

- **Community presence** means being seen in ordinary places that are typically shared by others in the community. Quality of life begins with being there in integrated and typical places and activities of everyday life.

- **Choice** is about having ample opportunities to direct one's life. It involves making decisions about both small and life-defining issues. Choice has often been used as a justification for segregation, implying that people with disabilities have chosen to be institutionalized, placed in group homes, or placed in sheltered facilities. However, when given opportunities to experience a typical lifestyle in the community, few choose segregation (Murphy et al., 2002).

- **Community participation** is being part of a growing network of personal relationships that provide opportunities for close friendships. Community participation means being a regular presence in everyday settings—being involved, getting to know others, and becoming known.

- **Respect** is having a valued place among a network of people and valued roles in everyday life. People gain respect through status-enhancing roles that are valued in our society such as worker, neighbor, friend, home owner, consumer, taxpayer, and volunteer.

• **Competence** is having the opportunity to perform activities that are meaningful and useful and building one's repertoire of skills and abilities in order to gain independence.

The impetus for this book stemmed from long-term interactions with a variety of stakeholders, including people with disabilities, family members, policy makers, state agency personnel, day and residential service providers, school personnel, and advocates. The book grew out of extensive work to investigate, promote, develop, monitor, and evaluate innovative services and supports for people with significant disabilities. It is an attempt to describe many of the innovations that have impacted changes at the federal, state, and local levels, and have resulted in quality outcomes for people with high support needs.

In our society, paid work is the anchor of most adults' days. Thus, a core component of this book is employment in regular businesses or entrepreneurial ventures. Yet, having a meaningful daytime is broader than just work—even for people who work full time, but especially for those who work only part time, or those who may not work at all. Meaningful daytimes may involve accessing community services, engaging in social and recreational activities, volunteering, furthering one's education, or pursuing other areas of interest. For example, Table 1.4 provides a listing of some of the many activities that typically comprise a meaningful day.

Table 1.4. Typical components of a meaningful day

Meaningful day activities	Examples
Work	✓ Exploring job options and opportunities ✓ Securing a job ✓ Starting your own business
Volunteer	✓ Meals on Wheels ✓ Survive Alive ✓ Food bank ✓ Church
Lifelong learning	✓ Taking adult education classes ✓ Attending a community college ✓ Receiving tutoring to build skills
Community involvement	✓ Joining community organizations ✓ Becoming a "regular" at a local establishment ✓ Using community services (bank, grocery, etc.)
Having fun and being social	✓ Using recreational facilities ✓ Attending movies, concerts, and performances ✓ Hanging out with friends ✓ Traveling

(continued)

Table 1.4. *(continued)*

Meaningful day activities	Examples
Health and wellness	✓ Exercising
	✓ Eating right
	✓ Monitoring one's health
Spirituality	✓ Going to church
	✓ Exploring one's beliefs
Housekeeping	✓ Cleaning
	✓ Cooking
	✓ House and yard maintenance

SUMMARY

The subsequent chapters in this book describe positive practices related to school to adult life transition, meaningful employment options, lifelong learning and adult education, community connections and relationships, advocacy and self-advocacy, retirement, organizational change, and future directions for policy and practice.

Readers are encouraged to ponder their own lives and the qualities that make them meaningful as they read this book. Ask why people with disabilities continue to face so many barriers to achieving meaningful daytimes. Analyze the many strategies that have helped individuals fulfill their dreams. Most importantly, determine what you and your counterparts will do as change agents to push for systems change.

REFERENCES

Americans with Disabilities Act of 1990, PL 101-336, 42 U.S.C. §§ 12101 *et seq.*

Architectural Barriers Act of 1968, PL 90-480, 42 U.S.C. §§ 4151 *et seq.*

Blatt, B., & Kaplan, F. (1974). *Christmas in purgatory: A photographic essay on mental retardation.* Syracuse, NY: Human Policy Press.

Braddock, D., Hemp, R., Rizzolo, M., Coulter, D., Haffer, L., & Thompson, M. (2005). *The state of the state in developmental disabilities 2005.* Washington, DC: American Association on Mental Retardation.

Bradley, V., Agosta, J., Taub, S., Smith, G., Taylor, M., Ashbaugh, J.W., et al. (2001). *The Robert Wood Johnson Foundation Self-Determination Initiative: Final impact assessment report.* Cambridge, MA: Human Services Research Institute.

Bradley, V.J. (1994). Evolution of a new service paradigm. In V.J. Bradley, J.W. Ashbaugh, & B.C. Blaney (Eds.), *Creating individual supports for people with developmental disabilities: A mandate for change at many levels.* Baltimore: Paul H. Brookes Publishing Co.

Carl D. Perkins Vocational and Applied Technology Education Act Amendments of 1990, PL 101-392, 104 Statutes at Large 753-804, 806-834.

Deutsch, A. (1948). *The shame of the state.* New York: Harcourt, Brace, and Company.

Developmental Disabilities Assistance and Bill of Rights Act of 1975, PL 94-103, 100 Stat. 840, 42 U.S.C. §§ 6000 *et seq.*

Education for All Handicapped Children Act of 1975, PL 94-142, 20 U.S.C. §§ 1400 *et seq.*

Education of the Handicapped Act of 1970, PL 91-230, 84 Stat. 121-154, 20 U.S.C. §§ 1400 *et seq.*

Fair Housing Act Amendments Act of 1988, PL 100-430, 42 U.S.C. §§ 3601 *et seq.*

Flynn, R., & Lemay, R. (1999). *A quarter-century of normalization and social role valorization: Evolution and impact.* Ottawa: University of Ottawa Press.

Fox-Grage, W., Folkemer, D., & Lewis, J. (2006). *The states' response to the Olmstead decision: How are states complying?* Washington, DC: National Council of State Legislatures.

Housing and Community Development Amendments of 1974, PL 93-383, 42 U.S.C. §§ 5309 *et seq.*

Individuals with Disabilities Education Act Amendments of 1991, PL 102-119, 20 U.S.C. §§ 1400 *et seq.*

Individuals with Disabilities Education Act Amendments of 1997, PL 105-17, 20 U.S.C. §§ 1400 *et seq.*

Individuals with Disabilities Education Improvement Act of 2004, PL 108-446, 20 U.S.C. §§ 1400 *et seq.*

Individuals with Disabilities Education Act of 1990, PL 101-476, 20 U.S.C. §§ 1400 *et seq.*

Kitchener, M., Willmott, M., Wong, A., & Harrington, C. (2006). *Home and community-based service: Introduction to Olmstead lawsuits and Olmstead plans.* San Francisco: UCSF National Center for Personal Assistance Services.

Kennedy, F. (1942). The problem of social control of the congenital defective: Education, sterilization, euthanasia. *American Journal of Psychiatry, 99,* 13–16.

Jackson, L. (2006). *Issues in severe disabilities.* Retrieved December 8, 2006, from http://www.unco.edu/nclid/SevereIssues.htm

Lakin, C., & Turnbull, A. (Eds.). (2005). *National goals and research for people with intellectual and developmental disabilities.* Washington, DC: The Arc of the United States and American Association on Mental Retardation.

Martin, E., Martin, R., & Terman, D. (1996). The legislative and litigation history of special education. *The Future of Children: Special Education for Students with Disabilities, 6*(1), 25–39.

Minnesota Governor's Council on Developmental Disabilities. (2006). *Parallels in time II.* St. Paul, MN: Author.

Murphy, S., Rogan, P., Handley, M., Kincaid, C., & Royce-Davis, J. (2002). People's situations and perspectives 8 years after workshop conversion. *Mental Retardation, 40*(1), 30–40.

Nirje, B. (1970). The normalization principle: Implications and comments. *Journal of Mental Retardation, 16,* 62–70.

O'Brien, J., & O'Brien, C.L. (1990). *A framework for accomplishment.* Decatur, GA: Responsive Systems Associates.

O'Brien, J. (1999). Education in applying the principle of normalization as a factor in the practical arts of improving services for people with disabilities. In R. Flynn & R. Lemay (Eds.), *A quarter-century of normalization and social role valorization: Evolution and impact.* Ottawa: University of Ottawa Press.

Olmstead v. L.C. and E.W., 527 U.S. 581; 119 S.Ct. 2176 (1990).

Prouty, R. & Lakin, C. (2005, September). Status of institutional closure efforts in 2005. *Policy Research Brief, 16*(1). Minneapolis: University of Minnesota Institute on Community Inclusion.

Racino, J. (Ed.). (1999). *Policy, program evaluation, and research in disability: Community support for all.* Binghamton, NY: The Haworth Press.

Rehabilitation Act Amendments of 1986, PL 99-506, 20 U.S.C. §§ 701 *et seq.*

Rehabilitation Act Amendments of 1992, PL 102-569, 29 U.S.C. §§ 701 *et seq.*

Rehabilitation Act of 1973, PL 93-112, 29 U.S.C. §§ 701 *et seq.*

Reid, D.H., Parsons, M.B., & Green, C.W. (2001). Evaluating the functional utility of congregate day treatment activities for adults with severe disabilities. *American Journal on Mental Retardation, 106*(5), 460–469.

Rizzolo, M.C., Hemp, R., Braddock, D., & Pomeranz-Essley, A. (2004). *The state of the states in developmental disabilities.* Washington, DC: American Association on Mental Retardation.

School-to-Work Opportunities Act of 1994, PL 103-239, 20 U.S.C. §§ 6101 *et seq.*

Social Security Act Amendments of 1967, PL 90-48, 42 U.S.C. §§ 1396 *et seq.*

Social Security Act Amendments of 1983, PL 98-21, 42 U.S.C. §§ 401 *et seq.*

Taylor, S. (1988). Caught in the continuum: A critical analysis of the principle of the least restrictive environment. *Journal of the Association for Persons with Severe Handicaps, 13*(1), 41–53.

Taylor, S.J. (1987). Continuum traps. In S. J. Taylor, D. Biklen, & J. Knoll (Eds.), *Community integration for people with severe disabilities* (pp. 25–35). New York: Teachers College Press.

Technology-Related Assistance for Individuals with Disabilities Act Amendments of 1994, PL 103-218, 29 U.S.C. §§ 2201 *et seq.*

Technology-Related Assistance for Individuals with Disabilities Act of 1988, PL 100-407, 29 U.S.C. §§ 2201 *et seq.*

Telecommunications for the Disabled Act of 1982, PL 97-410, 47 U.S.C. §§ 610 *et seq.*

Vail, D.J., & Thomas, C.C. (1966). Dehumanization and the institutional career. *Hospital Community Psychiatry, 17,* 367–377.

Vocational Education Act of 1963, PL 88-210, 20 U.S.C. §§ 35 *et seq.*

Wolfensberger, W. (1972). *The principle of normalization in human services.* Toronto: National Institute on Mental Retardation.

CHAPTER TWO

Preparing for Meaningful Adult Lives Through School and Transition Experiences

PATRICIA ROGAN, RICHARD LUECKING, AND TERESA GROSSI

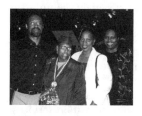

Throughout the nation, three circumstances typically distinguish youth with significant disabilities from their typically developing peers. First, they are likely to be educated in segregated self-contained classrooms and settings, apart from their peers who do not receive special education services. This is in spite of the Individuals with Disabilities Education Improvement Act (IDEA) of 2004 (PL 108-446) that states that children are to be educated within the general education setting with appropriate services and supports brought in, unless it can be proven that they are unable to learn in this environment. There is a growing body of research that shows the mutual benefits of inclusive education to both students with and without disability labels (Burstein, Sears, Wilcoxen, Cabello, & Schalock, 2004; Friend & Bursuck, 2002; Lipsky & Gartner, 1995; Manset & Semmel, 1997; McDonnell et al., 2003; Ryndak, Jackson, & Billingsley, 1999–2000; Salend, 1999). Although many educators attempt to teach functional skills in self-contained settings, students with significant disabilities are often engaged in activities that are neither meaningful nor preparatory.

Second, students with significant disabilities typically remain in high school after age 18, when their peers without disabilities have moved on to postsecondary educational settings and employment (Neubert, Moon, & Grigal, 2002). In fact, many students spend 8 or more years within the confines of a high school building before exiting the public schools. Although a portion of their school day may involve non–school instruction in community, employment, and recreational settings, their daily schedule, the people they are with, and the attitudes and expectations of educators and parents during this time typically reflect a school day and student status rather than an adult's day in the real world.

Third, contrary to almost all of their peers without disabilities, students with significant disabilities will have fewer prospects as adults of achieving employment in integrated, direct-hire jobs; living in a home of their own; gaining access to an array of community services; and engaging in satisfying social relationships and activities. According to the National Transition Longitudinal Study–2 (2005) of more than 8,000 students who received special education services, 48.9% of graduates were working full time, most in low-wage, low-status jobs, with few opportunities for advancement. Employment outcomes for youth with significant disabilities are even worse. Most end up in segregated, congregate day activity programs or sheltered workshops (Butterworth, Gilmore, Kiernan, & Schalock, 1999; Rizzolo, Hemp, Braddock, & Pomeranz-Essley, 2004). Unfortunately, even students who have had job training in school may fall through the cracks due to multiple factors, including poor transition planning, waiting lists, lack of sufficient funding for ongoing supports, or other difficulties with our complex and disjointed adult service system.

Segregated educational services, curriculum that is not preparatory, inconsistent linkages with adult service agencies, underfunded and inadequate adult services, and adult unemployment and segregation remain the unfortunate status quo for most individuals with significant disabilities. Fortunately, there are many effective approaches that have been implemented to address these circumstances. Many youth with high support needs have successful educational, transition, and adult experiences. The purpose of this chapter is to describe an array of educational and transition practices that can positively impact the postschool outcomes of youth with significant disabilities. The chapter begins with a brief description of the evolution of transition services. Next, general features of effective educational practices are summarized. The chapter then highlights some of the major issues and practices related to transition services. The next section focuses on specific secondary education practices that have proven successful in preparing youth and their families for adult life: student-centered planning and a focus on self-determination, inclusive high school opportunities, off-campus transition services, and interagency collaboration and funding. The chapter concludes with recommendations and future directions.

THE EVOLUTION OF TRANSITION PRACTICES

The field of special education has evolved tremendously in terms of values and practices in the past 2 decades. The authors began their professional careers when students were served in segregated schools or were just beginning to be served in public schools (but often in the basement or the far wing of a school). In the 1980s, progressive school services for youth with significant disabilities involved instruction in functional life domains (e.g., vocational, domestic, community, recreation/leisure). Through community-based instruction and job training, students spent a great deal of time away from the school building. At that time, community-based instruction began in elementary school and job training began as early as middle school for many students (Brown et al., 1983;

Falvey, 1986). At the time, many students were merely visitors in public schools, with minimal connections to the life of the school.

The mid-1980s through the present day brought an orientation toward inclusive education and, with it, an understanding that the public school represents students' community more than the larger community outside the school building for elementary and middle school students. Rather than pull students out of school buildings during the day to receive instruction in the community, the Individuals with Disabilities Education Act (IDEA) Amendments of 1997 (PL 105-17) called for involvement in general education settings and activities to the maximum extent possible with appropriate services and supports brought in. Practices such as co-planning and co-teaching (Friend & Bursuck, 2001), cooperative learning (Villa, Thousand, Nevin, & Liston, 2005), peer buddies (Hughes et al., 2000), individualized adaptations, assistive technology and accommodations, and differentiated instruction (Tomlinson, Stronge, & Cunningham-Eidson, 2003) have emerged to support inclusive education.

Supported employment, which targeted people with severe disabilities, emerged in the early 1980s (Gold, 1980). In 1986, the Rehabilitation Act Amendments (PL 99-506) recognized supported employment as a legitimate outcome of the vocational rehabilitation (VR) system for the first time. Supported employment provides individualized job development, on-the-job training or consultation, and ongoing support services to individuals who have typically been excluded from the workforce to work in typical job settings. Support to get and keep employment has allowed people with significant disabilities to work in integrated community businesses.

As discussed in Chapter 1, federal legislation has served to guide state and local policies and practices. The passage of IDEA in 1990 required transition planning and services for youth with disabilities. Such plans, referred to as individualized transition plans (ITPs), were required as part of the individualized education program (IEP). The IDEA Amendments of 1997 stated that by the age of 14 (or earlier, if appropriate), IEPs shall include a statement of the student's transition service needs, based on career considerations and focused on the student's courses of study. By the age of 16, the transition component of the IEP should emphasize the necessary linkages with other agencies and programs in the school and community that can affect transition outcomes in the different goal areas.

The most recent reauthorization of IDEA, referred to as IDEA 2004, defines transition as

1. Designed to be within a results-oriented process, that is focused on improving the academic and functional achievement of the child with a disability to facilitate the child's movement from school to postschool activities including postsecondary education, vocational education, integrated employment (including supported employment), continuing and adult education, adult services, independent living, or community participation;

2. Is based on the individual child's needs, taking into account the child's strengths, preferences, and interests, and includes a) training and education, b) related services, c) community experiences, c) the development of

employment and other postschool adult living objectives, and if appropriate, d) the acquisition of daily living skills and functional vocational evaluation.

Unfortunately, IDEA 2004 dropped the requirement to begin transition planning at age 14. Current language states that transition planning should begin no later than the first IEP that is in effect when the child turns 16, or younger if determined appropriate by the IEP team and updated annually thereafter. This change is unfortunate because the age 14 mandate provided the opportunity for school teams and families to plan for relevant and meaningful high school curricula and experiences to prevent school dropout for some students. Transition IEPs must now include

1. Appropriate measurable postsecondary goals based upon age-appropriate transition assessments related to training, education, employment, and where appropriate, independent living skills, and

2. The transition services (including courses of study) needed to assist the child in reaching those goals.

The Rehabilitation Act Amendments of 1986, now incorporated within the Workforce Investment Act (WIA) of 1998 (PL 105-220), govern VR programs at the federal and state levels, which provide employment services for eligible individuals with disabilities. WIA is linked with IDEA through a common definition of transition services. This is significant because the two Acts clearly promote collaboration and coordination between school and vocational rehabilitation services on behalf of students with disabilities in transition. WIA is a comprehensive job-training bill that consolidated previous federally funded programs at the federal, state, and local levels. The centerpiece of the WIA is a system of One-Stop centers designed to provide job training, education, and employment services in a single location. The key idea behind WIA is that every individual, including every individual with disabilities, has the right to gain access to the basic services that include three types or levels of services:

- Core services—including work exploration, job search skills training, interviewing techniques workshops, resume development, and referral to an employer with a position available

- Intensive services—for individuals who are unable to obtain employment by using the core services

- Training services—for individuals who do not become successfully employed by using the core and intensive services

Access to each level depends on the needs of the individual. Students in transition can take advantage of core services while they are in high school if educators share this information and facilitate the process. In addition, because VR is a required partner in the One-Stop delivery system, students can complete the referral process to VR at the One-Stop center. Partnerships between the One-Stop centers, VR services, and public schools should help youth and adults with disabilities to improve their employment outcomes.

Taken together, all of these pieces of legislation promote equal access and individualized, integrated services, and supports. The fields of special education and rehabilitation continue to evolve in all areas, with a growing emphasis on self-determination, empowerment, choice and control, self-advocacy, equal access, and individualized or customized services.

TRANSITIONS ACROSS THE LIFESPAN

Transitions—or the progression from one age period, developmental level, program, or setting, to another—can be stressful, even when the transitions are planned and smooth. Fear and stress stem from moving from what is familiar and comfortable to what is unknown. Although this chapter focuses on transition from school to work and adult life, it is important to understand that transition planning begins at a young age and continues across the lifespan. That is, when students move from early childhood to preschool services, from preschool to elementary school, elementary to middle, and middle to high school, transition planning must occur. This brief section highlights several important elements of these lifespan transitions, which set the tone and provide the foundation for school to adult life transition.

Longitudinal Alignment of Curriculum

Current state and national standards serve to align curriculum within public schools. However, teachers of students with more significant disabilities have traditionally operated outside of these standards. Furthermore, curricular approaches for students with high support needs often vary widely, even in the same school district. For example, an elementary teacher may have a self-contained classroom and focus on functional life domain areas, while the middle school teacher promotes inclusive education, and the high school teacher provides primarily community-based instruction. This lack of longitudinal alignment of the curriculum impedes student learning and can be very frustrating to families as they experience the lack of continuity. Special education services within school districts must be aligned philosophically and practically so that they systematically lead to desired outcomes.

Now, with the No Child Left Behind (NCLB) Act of 2001 (PL 107-110), all teachers are being held accountable for addressing state standards and participating in state assessments based on these standards. For teachers of students with significant disabilities, the question of how best to do this presents opportunities and challenges. On one hand, the focus on a uniform set of standards for all students may offer incentives for inclusive education where there was resistance in the past. However, the pressures associated with the requirements of NCLB (e.g., annual yearly progress, high stakes testing) may actually impede inclusive education as schools blame their failure to make annual yearly progress on students with disabilities, and as general education teachers retreat to a "skill and drill" approach to teaching. In the context of transition planning, special education teachers of students with significant disabilities struggle with how best to promote inclusive education, address meaningful life skills, and still adhere to the standards.

Annual Transition Planning from a Young Age

Year after year, students with significant disabilities move from school to
school and class to class with little or no preplanning and preparation. It is critical that sending and receiving teachers meet with family members to plan for
each transition. Sending teachers (e.g., those in middle school whose students
are moving on to high school) and receiving teachers (e.g., high school teachers who will serve these students the following year) need to meet to discuss
their curriculum, expectations, and practices so students can be prepared to
move smoothly from one level to the next. This can be facilitated by holding
IEP case conference meetings at the receiving school to give students and parents an opportunity to meet other team members. Team members should communicate strategies, materials, and specific accommodations and adaptations
that have been successful. Students should be given opportunities to visit their
new school, as needed, so they feel comfortable with the building, using a
locker, negotiating the lunchroom, changing classes, and so on.

Students should also participate in typical orientation activities with their
general education peers. Mentor relationships can be set up with peers to
smooth these transitions even further.

EFFECTIVE PRACTICES THAT PREPARE YOUTH AND THEIR FAMILIES FOR TRANSITION TO MEANINGFUL ADULT LIVES

Within the context of a lifespan approach to transition from school to adult life,
it is important to identify effective practices from elementary school through
high school that result in meaningful adult outcomes. Preparation for adult
roles encompasses employment, postsecondary education, lifelong learning,
community living in a typical home, use of community services, participation
in community activities, pursuit of personal interests during free time, and satisfying social relationships. Although decisions must always be based on the
unique needs of each student, the following section highlights essential components of an inclusive, preparatory education designed to lead to meaningful
adult outcomes for youth with significant disabilities.

Age-Appropriate and Inclusive Environments

Schools are a microcosm of our communities and should prepare all children
to live together in our diverse society. Being with same-age peers in inclusive
environments has provided valuable peer models for students with significant
disabilities. Students are more likely to be engaged in age-appropriate activities when they are educated with their same-age peers (Bennett, Deluca, &
Bruns, 1997; McDonnell, Hardman, Hightower, & Kiefer-O'Donnell, 1991).
Inclusive environments typically foster higher expectations and performance,
independence, and positive relationships with peers (Corbett, 2001; Fisher,
Roach, & Frey, 2002; Sands, Kozleski, & French, 2000) while resulting in the

same or improved academic performance by students without disabilities (Holahan & Costanbader, 2000; Kluth, Straut, & Biklen, 2003). Furthermore, once they get to know students with disabilities, both youth and adults in general education settings learn and grow in their understanding and attitudes. This is an important first step in preparing the next generation of parents, educators, employers, co-workers, neighbors, and community leaders to think and act differently.

Some believe that students with significant disabilities cannot learn functional life skills while receiving an inclusive education. In reality, exclusion from general education settings and activities denies students access to the attributes and skills related to success in today's world that *all* students need to 1) identify, organize, plan, and allocate resources; 2) work with others; 3) acquire and use information; 4) understand interrelationships; 5) work with a variety of technologies; 6) perform basic skills (e.g., read, write, listen, speak); 7) perform thinking skills (e.g., make decisions, solve problems, think creatively); and 8) display personal qualities (e.g., responsibility, self-esteem, self-management, sociability, honesty) (Kluth et al., 2003; U.S. Department of Labor, 1991). The success of inclusive education depends less on students' abilities than the attitudes, creativity, and collaboration of adults.

In addition to inclusive activities during the school day, students should have access to and support for participating in extracurricular activities. Not only do these activities provide another outlet for the development of social skills and relationships, they also provide a variety of leisure and career exploration opportunities (Bauer, 2001).

SELF-DETERMINATION: STUDENT INVOLVEMENT IN LIFE PLANNING

One of the primary roles of a public school education is to prepare youth to be responsible, contributing, and self-sufficient adults. Becoming self-determined is a lifelong process that must begin at a young age. Students with significant disabilities are often denied opportunities and experiences to develop self-determination skills due to overprotective adults, low expectations, negative attitudes, inadequate support, lack of choice- and decision-making opportunities, and lack of access to typical life opportunities (Wehmeyer, 1996; 2001).

Self-determination involves self-awareness (knowing one's strengths and needs), making choices and decisions that affect one's life, advocating for oneself, seeking assistance as needed, and being responsible for one's decisions (Wehmeyer, Palmer, Agran, Mithaug, & Martin, 2000). Since these are sophisticated skills that develop over time with experience and maturity, it is imperative to begin very early to address them. Infusing and emphasizing self-determination skills throughout the day and curriculum may require a major shift in the attitudes and practices of parents and educators (Thoma, Baker, & Saddler, 2002). Efforts must be made to put students in age-appropriate decision-making roles whereby students learn from their decisions (both good and bad), even when adults may disagree with particular decisions (Held, Thoma, & Thomas, 2004). Parents and educators can assist students to gradually assume more and more responsibilities at home and at school, solve minor and more complex problems, advocate for themselves, request help or advice when needed, and ultimately steer the direction of their lives. The following example illustrates how one teacher has worked to facilitate self-determination skills with her high school students and involve them in their own life planning.

STUDENT INVOLVEMENT IN TRANSITION PLANNING

Karen knew her high school–age students needed to be involved in their own life planning. How could she infuse development of self-advocacy and self-determination skills into the transition process? At first she began by having a set time during the school day when students partnered with peers without disabilities to identify postschool plans and action steps. She soon realized that efforts to increase student involvement, including choice making and decision making, needed to be embedded throughout the day and week. Yet some students with high support needs had difficulty with the abstract nature of planning for their future.

With the assistance of school and university personnel with expertise and creative ideas about technology, Karen began to use PowerPoint software with her students. The students began to use photos, videotape clips, and music to develop PowerPoint presentations, with adult and peer assistance, that depicted their current daily schedule, likes and dislikes, and desired next steps. In fact, Karen used the Next S.T.E.P. curriculum (Halpern, Herr, Doren, & Wolf, 2000) as a framework for planning with her students. The curriculum addresses domains of daily life, including work, home living, social/recreation, and community. By seeing visual depictions of current and future lifestyles, students have begun to better understand and advocate more strongly for what they want.

Student involvement in transition planning has evolved to the point where all her students lead their transition conferences. They share their individually designed PowerPoint presentations with team members at their transition meetings and ask for input and support to reach their goals. Even students who do not talk or who have limited communication skills can share their "voice" through this technology. One example of the powerful impact of this approach involves a young man we will call Kevin. Kevin expressed his desire to live in his own apartment. After he got a job, Kevin's circle of support assisted him to move into his own place prior to exit from high school. Now other students want what Kevin has! Student voices continue to be strengthened through their active involvement in, and self-direction of, transition planning.

PERSON-CENTERED PLANNING AND TRANSITION

Individualized, or person-centered, planning forms the foundation of educational services for youth with disabilities. Such plans are based on the notion of starting with the end in mind. That is, teams must use backward planning as they develop IEPs and deliver services and supports in order to increase the likelihood that desired outcomes are achieved. John and Connie Lyle O'Brien's *A Framework for Accomplishment* (1990), described in Chapter 1, can be used as a focal point of person-centered planning. Quality of life depends on community presence (regular physical presence in a variety of typical community settings), choice (control over one's life), competence (gaining skills, abilities, and independence), respect (valued community roles), and community participation (involvement in meaningful, inclusive activities and a network of personal relationships). Person-centered planning tools, such as PATH (Pearpoint, O'Brien, & Forest, 1993) and personal futures planning (Mount, 2000), can be used effectively for transition planning with transition teams. Although a thorough description of person-centered planning approaches is beyond the scope of this chapter, the various processes typically involve discussions about questions such as:

- What is your vision for the future (employment, living, social/recreation, community, postsecondary education)?
- What are the student's strengths/gifts/talents/capacities?
- What are the student's interests and preferences?
- What are the student's challenges and support needs?
- What actions should be taken to move toward achieving the vision?
- Who will undertake these actions and by when?

Maps, or visual depictions of the responses to these questions (e.g., using chart paper, markers, colorful graphics) are typically used to display this information. Ideally, the information that is generated is captured and shared in writing and ultimately used to guide transition planning.

Traditionally, transition and IEP planning processes have been fraught with difficulties that impede the involvement of students and parents (Kyeong Hwa & Turnbull, 2004). As noted by Thoma, Rogan, and Baker (2001), students are often excluded from IEP and transition planning meetings. Even parents are often relegated to passive roles as recipients of information from school and adult service personnel. Logistical problems (e.g., little time for good discussion and decision making at meetings, IEPs already written prior to case conference meetings) also impede thorough planning. Individualized backward planning (or personal futures planning) should begin with families when their child is in preschool. Although it may be difficult for some parents to take a lead role on a planning team, it is important that they be central to the process. After all, most parents will continue to be the primary advocate and support provider for their children until they are adults. At times, parents or guardians may struggle to envision a positive future for their child. Educators can assist parents by providing information and resources, linking parents with other parents, and describing a vision of an inclusive adult lifestyle. Sometimes family members need to assist school personnel to adopt a positive vision of the future for a particular student. Students should be involved in case conference meetings and informal planning sessions to the maximum extent possible throughout their school careers. Parent empowerment is as important as student empowerment during the transition process, enabling parents to negotiate the adult service maze, and to facilitate natural supports.

PARENT INVOLVEMENT AND EMPOWERMENT

There is a strong correlation between parent involvement in IEP planning and support of educational activities, and postschool success (Epstein et al., 2002; Morningstar & Torrez, 2003; Wandry & Pleet, 2003). Parents often express frustration about the format of transition planning meetings, especially if insufficient time has been allotted for discussion, if mandated forms have already been completed without parental input, if the forms themselves do not adequately capture the student's transition needs and preferences, if the parent feels overwhelmed by the volume of information that is shared, and/or if the parents' questions cannot be answered.

Schools can promote parental involvement by sharing critical information about school and adult services in user-friendly and alternative formats. For example, the following options might be developed for sharing information with families:

- One-page summaries of important topics such as Medicaid waivers (e.g., types and how to apply), accessible transportation options, each of the state agencies (e.g., Developmental Disabilities, Mental Health), Social Security (including how and where to apply for SSI and work incentives information), obtaining an identification card, and age of majority/guardianship issues and actions
- A videotape summary of the transition process and actions that families should take, including timelines
- A web site that contains the information stated above
- Periodic parent meetings with guest speakers (e.g., state funding agency personnel, adult service providers, parents of young adults who have already made the transition out of school)
- Transition fairs where multiple agencies and services are represented in one place, allowing families to speak directly with individuals and gather information

CAREER EXPLORATION AND JOB TRAINING

The primary purpose of career exploration is to provide students with an array of work-related opportunities to demonstrate skills in the actual settings in which they will be used (i.e., real work setting) to 1) determine their strengths, abilities, interests, and support and accommodation needs; 2) analyze the environment, including job skills and work-related requirements; and 3) match the information based on the student and the environment to make a job match. From an education standpoint, the focus should be on 1) assessment and instruction, not development of proficiency in a single job, and 2) gaining sufficient information to lead to an "ideal" job match. While on the various job sites, the role of school personnel is essential. For some programs, such as work-study programs, students are paid and considered employees of the company. For other programs, like community-based vocational training programs, U.S. Department of Labor regulations must be consulted to ensure that students are performing like trainees and not employees.

Students with disabilities are more likely to make smooth transitions to adult work if they have had real work experiences during high school (Wehman, 2006). This factor is perhaps the strongest link to postschool employment success, as various studies have shown the value of paid work experiences in high school as predictors of later adult employment success (Luecking & Fabian, 2000; Phelps & Hanley-Maxwell, 1997).

NATURAL WORKPLACE SUPPORTS

Schools are typically richer in resources than adult services. Schools may opt to provide one-to-one assistance for particular students or assign job coaches to work individually with students at job sites. While such support may be necessary for some students, it is imperative that school staff understand the importance of fading their support and facilitating the involvement of natural supports whenever possible. Having a school staff person constantly at the student's side (the "bodyguard" approach) may build in dependence on the part of the student, may repel peers and coworkers without disabilities, and may send a message that only "special" people can provide support. Overreliance on one-to-one support also fosters dependence on the part of employers, and may prevent them from taking ownership of, and responsibility for, the student.

Studies about workplace supports have demonstrated the importance of adhering to typical business practices and promoting the involvement of workplace personnel in order to benefit the supported employee (Mank, Cioffi, & Yovanoff, 2000; Rogan, Banks, & Howard, 2001). Job coaches need to be aware of workplace cultures, including typical rituals, routines, and practices, in order to assist supported employees to blend in and develop relationships with coworkers. Job coaches should not take over job training and support functions, but should facilitate the capacity of workplace personnel to provide support. If direct job coach interventions are required, they should be provided discreetly, while adhering to the norms of the workplace, and involving coworkers as much as possible.

TRANSITION SERVICES FOR YOUTH AGES 18–21

Off-campus (totally nonschool) transition services for youth between the ages of 18 and 21 are an ideal way for students to experience graduation and continue to receive school-funded support to experience typical adult settings and activities. Many versions of nonschool, community-based services for youth ages 18–21 exist throughout the country. Some areas have opted to develop a formal program on community college or university campuses, while others simulate typical adult schedules and activities. These two options are described below.

THE BALTIMORE TRANSITION CONNECTION

One such program called the Baltimore Transition Connection, has been established by the Baltimore City Public School system (BCPSS) (Grigal, Divyre, & Davis, 2006). Local school districts typically enter into a cooperative agreement with the postsecondary institution that allows students the use of college space and facilities in return for any number of remunerated and in-kind benefits. The major benefit to the school system is that it is able to expand and improve relevant services to young adults so that they are better prepared for postschool life. As of this writing, BCPSS is delivering educational services to 30 students between the ages of 18 and 21 with significant disabilities in cooperation with three postsecondary educational institutions: Baltimore City Community College, Coppin State University, and The Johns Hopkins University. These students are not projected to receive a regular high school diploma and most were previously receiving educational services in segregated special education schools. Each of these campuses hosts 10 students. College students are recruited to provide volunteer support to students as they participate in campus life.

Young adults in programs located on campuses typically receive a combination of classroom and community-based instruction of functional and life skills, paid and unpaid employment experiences, use of campus facilities (e.g., library, career center, fitness center), participation in clubs or activities on campus, and participation in college courses—usually by audit. Individual interests, needs, and IEP goals determine the percentage of the day spent on each of these activities.

Teachers and other educational staff organize and deliver instruction so that the students spend their days on the college campus or on community work sites. A critical benefit of this approach is the opportunity for students to interact and spend time with students without disabilities on the campus, thus learning social behaviors and establishing typical friendships. Just as critical is the time spent in campus community work environments where they learn job behaviors and skills that will benefit their career development. The primary objective of these programs is for students to exit mandated publicly supported education with a meaningful and productive lifestyle, including employment, lifelong learning, community access and involvement, social opportunities, and other individually desirable aspects of life.

The features of the Baltimore Transition Connection include

- Instruction that is entirely community based in age-appropriate environments, including community and four-year colleges as well as worksites throughout the Baltimore community

- Highly individualized activities and supports based on the IEP and person-centered assessment. Schedules and learning opportunities are designed as a result of comprehensive student assessment and input.

- Highly contextual teaching, emphasizing community experiences, especially those that are work-based. All students participate in at least one paid work experience during their time in the program, and most have several work experiences.

- Collaborative instruction whereby BCPSS teachers and staff work in close association with adult agency staff who will serve the students upon exit from school services. At least 6 months prior to school exit, personnel from adult agencies selected by the student and his/her family will begin providing support to students through a cooperative arrangement with the schools.

"TYPICAL DAY" TRANSITION SERVICES

Another approach to graduation and post–high school experiences has been demonstrated by several high schools in Indiana. Students are not automatically based at a college or university and they are never all grouped together. Instead, youth design their individualized daily schedule with their person-centered team (or circle of support) based on their desired adult lifestyle. Students begin and end their days at their homes, while engaging in a variety of employment, postsecondary education, community, recreational, and social activities during the day and week. Like the BCPSS program described above, the goal of this effort is to establish reliable, affordable, and typical transportation options, secure gainful employment, develop daily and weekly routines during non-work times with needed supports (e.g., taking a class; exercising; meeting friends; going to a bank, restaurant, or store) for each student prior to official school exit. A representative weekly schedule is shown in Figure 2.1.

Adult service personnel may be involved anytime between the ages of 18–21, depending on the agency and specific service, and the student's timeline for formal school exit.

SCHOOL–BUSINESS PARTNERSHIPS

In order to create successful school–business partnerships, each partner needs to learn how to work together and understand each other's needs and requirements. Employers can become involved with schools in a variety of ways while understanding that their contributions are preparing the future workforce. The National Employer Leadership Council (1996) published the Employer Participation Model that offers a variety of opportunities for employers to partner with schools.

- Career talks—visit the classroom and share information about the business and industry

- Career fairs—attend special events to allow students to meet with employers and ask questions about different industries

- Workplace and industry tours—host student visits during which they talk to employees and observe workplace activities

- Job shadowing—arrange for students to follow an employee at a business to learn about a specific occupation or industry

- Job rotations—arrange for students to transfer among a variety of positions and tasks requiring different skills and responsibilities to understand all the steps in a product or service

- Internships—employ students for a specified period of time so they can learn about a specific industry or occupation

- Cooperative education—arrange for students to alternate or coordinate their high school studies with a job in a field related to their academic or occupational objective

- Youth apprenticeships—combine school- and work-based learning over multiple years in a specific occupational area or cluster designed to lead directly into a related postsecondary program, entry-level job, or registered apprenticeship program

- Mentoring—pair students with employers who instruct the students, critique performance, challenge them to perform well, and who work in consultation with teachers

Each of these potential employer activities present important options for educators and transition specialists to link students with critical work-based learning opportunities. Locating good employment opportunities is essential for all students to be successful. School personnel, usually the transition coordinator or work-study coordinator, must have a clear understanding of the ever-changing expectations and demands of the workplace and the role of the student. School personnel must leave the school world and enter the business world. To do this, a number of areas must be addressed:

1. Businesses are concerned about the student attending as scheduled and performing their job duties. The work must be performed around the needs and hours of operation of the business, not the school hours or school schedule. For example, students may be required to work during a holiday break or throughout the summer. Schools will need to make the appropriate arrangements to assure proper supports.

2. Each workplace is different and each requires different expectations for work and social performance. Schools must have a clear understanding of appropriate and acceptable performance in the workplace. For example, there are some students who like to hug the teacher in the morning. Although hugging friends is acceptable, in a workplace this could be misconstrued as sexual harassment.

	Monday	Tuesday	Wednesday	Thursday	Friday
8:00	Take bus at 8:15 to 4th and Washington Walk to Bakehouse restaurant	Take bus at 8:15 to 4th and Washington Walk to Bakehouse restaurant	Take bus at 8:15 to 4th and Washington Walk to Bakehouse restaurant	Take bus at 8:15 to 4th and Washington Walk to Bakehouse restaurant	Take bus at 8:15 to 4th and Washington Walk to Bakehouse restaurant
9:00	Work	Work	Work	Work	Work
10:00	Work	Work	Work	Work	Work
11:00	Work	Work	Work	Work	Work
12:00	Work	Work	Work	Work	Work
1:00	Lunch with Lauren #3 bus to the YMCA	Bring lunch Walk to the library Eat at the library Check e-mail	Bring lunch Walk to City Hall Eat at City Hall Check e-mail	Bring lunch Walk to the library Eat at the library Check e-mail	Respite pick-up Lunch at home
1:30	YMCA	Library	Volunteer job at City Hall	Library	Weekly errands
2:30	YMCA	Adult education class at university	Volunteer	Adult education class at university	Weekly errands
3:00	Respite person meets at YMCA or at home. (Every other week meet friend at his apartment at 3:30)	Class	Respite person meets at City Hall	Class	
Evenings		Self-advocates group 4th Tuesday, 5:30–7:00 Unitarian Church Spend night with Mom	Evening with Dad		Every other weekend with Dad

Figure 2.1. Sample weekly schedule for community-based transition services for youth ages 18–21.

3. Most companies are more than willing to partner with schools to assist in their future workforce. However, schools must also be sensitive to the fact that a business must continue to operate and make a profit, therefore not requiring an extensive additional amount of work.

4. Watch the language! School personnel are ambassadors for their schools and students. Businesses tend to be concerned with getting the job done and what can be contributed to the business. Care should be given to speaking about students with respect and dignity while not using labels or disclosing personal information. Interactions should focus on the strengths of the individuals and his or her individual experiences and/or contributions.

INTERAGENCY COLLABORATION AND INNOVATIVE FUNDING

Interagency collaboration and individualized, sufficient funding are essential to promoting a seamless transition from school to meaningful adult lives, and for preventing students from falling through the cracks between school entitlement and eligibility-based adult services (Luecking & Certo, 2002; Kohler, 2003). School and adult services can appear to be worlds apart in terms of entitlement (or lack thereof), eligibility, funding, service coordination, and practices. Both school personnel and family members are often uninformed and confused about adult services. Adult service personnel are often overwhelmed with their caseloads, and may not communicate with schools in a coordinated and timely fashion. One approach to facilitating interagency collaboration is to form a community transition council comprised of key stakeholder group representatives. Such a group can include the school transition coordinator and/or vocational staff, parents, students in transition, employers, adult service agencies (e.g., residential, employment), state funding agencies (e.g., developmental disabilities, VR, mental health), and other key players (e.g., independent living, case managers, university personnel). Community transition councils can address such issues as interagency agreements between schools and adult services, business partnerships, transition services activities, expectations, and timelines, transition materials such as brochures and booklets, and training needs such as workshops and conferences.

Another approach is to integrate the resources of the school, vocational rehabilitation, and adult service providers during the last year of the student's publicly supported education (Luecking & Certo, 2002). In this transition model the student's last year of school is organized around individually determined jobs and community activities that will ideally be part of the student's postschool adult life. School personnel and adult service agency personnel work collaboratively to help the student find employment and engage in desired community activities such as going to the gym or pursuing other meaningful adult oriented activities. The involvement of the adult agency is to ensure a seamless transition with job and community supports in place upon school exit. This approach is made possible through innovative braiding of school system, vocational rehabilitation, and developmental disabilities agency funds and resources, whereby each system agrees to commit resources during the final year in school to enable this seamless transition. The intended result is that the first day after school exit looks no different to the youth than the last day of school; working in the same job and participating in the same community activities, with the same people available for supporting them for long-term employment success and community participation.

GRADUATE FOLLOW-UP STUDIES

Graduate follow-up studies allow the sending agencies or the school to track the status and outcomes of youth with disabilities who have left school and entered the adult world. Follow-up studies allow schools to ask the basic question of "How well are we preparing students for life after high school?" Typically, postsecondary outcome information is gathered on the employment status (i.e., full time, part time, salary, time of job, how the job was found), postsecondary education status (i.e., attending college/university, community college, vocational/technical college), residential status (i.e., living alone or with family), personal/social status (i.e., leisure and recreation activities, relationships, friendships, and overall quality of life issues), and access to community resources (i.e., VR services, workforce development offices, developmental disabilities, or mental health services).

Follow-along studies gather data on youth with disabilities over an extended period of time whereas follow-up studies gather data on a single occasion after a predetermined period of time has elapsed. Regardless of the approach, it is important for school personnel to gather essential information to be used to 1) promote a smooth transfer for youth with disabilities from school to postschool environments, 2) promote quality postsecondary outcomes for youth with disabilities, and 3) evaluate the overall quality of the transition program and services provided to youth with disabilities.

SUMMARY

Although much progress has been made, many challenges remain to preparing all youth for meaningful adult lives through school and transition experiences. This chapter highlighted the importance of educating youth with disabilities in inclusive settings to the maximum extent possible, and providing a preparatory curriculum that starts with the end in mind. Students need to be supported from a young age to develop self-determination skills and to be active participants in their educational and life planning. Person-centered planning approaches have proven to be very effective for backwards planning. By beginning with a vision of a desirable future and taking a strengths-based approach, team members can work together to achieve desired outcomes. An essential component of a preparatory education is career development experiences and job training activities. Real jobs in integrated settings with decent wages and benefits must be the focus. The process of facilitating internal, or natural, supports within businesses is a key strategy to ensure employment success.

Another critical transition strategy is to capitalize on the final 3 years of a student's high school education to provide intensive transition services. Strategies for nonschool, community-based transition services for youth ages 18–21 were offered. In addition, the need for interagency collaboration and innovative funding was emphasized. We must continue to track the outcomes of public school graduates (including those who do not receive a diploma) in order to monitor progress and make improvements. After up to 18 years of a public school education, students with disabilities deserve a decent quality of life as adults.

REFERENCES

Bauer, A. (2001). *Adolescents and inclusion: Transforming secondary schools.* Baltimore: Paul H. Brookes Publishing Co.

Bennett, T., DeLuca, D., & Bruns, D. (1997). Putting inclusion into practice: Perspectives of teachers and parents. *Exceptional Children, 64*(1), 115–131.

Brown, L., Shiraga, B., Ford, A., Nisbet, J., VanDeventer, P., Sweet, et al. (1983). Teaching severely handicapped students to perform meaningful work in nonsheltered vocational environments. In L. Brown, A. Ford, J. Nisbet, M. Sweet, B. Shiraga, J. York, et al. (Eds.), *Educational programs for severely handicapped students* (vol. XIII). Madison, WI: Madison Metropolitan School District.

Burstein, N., Sears, S., Wilcoxen, A., Cabello, B., & Spagna, M. (2004). Moving toward inclusive practices, *Remedial & Special Education, 25*(2), 104–116.

Butterworth, J., Gilmore, D., Kiernan, W., & Schalock, R. (1999). *State trends in employment services for people with developmental disabilities: Multiyear comparisons based on state mental retardation/developmental disability agency and vocational rehabilitation data.* Boston: Institute for Community Inclusion, Children's Hospital.

Corbett, J. (2001). *Supporting inclusive education: A connective pedagogy.* London and New York: Routledge.

Epstein, J., Jansom, N., Salinas, K., Sanders, M., & Van Vorhis, F. (2002). *School, family, and community partnerships: Your handbook for action.* Thousand Oaks, CA: Sage Publishing.

Falvey, M.A. (1986). Community skills. In M.A. Falvey, *Community-based curriculum: Instructional strategies for students with severe handicaps* (pp. 61–76). Baltimore: Paul H. Brookes Publishing Co.

Fisher, D., Roach, V., & Frey, N. (2002). Examining the general programmatic benefits of inclusive schools. *International Journal of Inclusive Education, 6*(1), 63–78.

Friend, M., & Bursuck, W.D. (2001). *Including students with special needs: A practical guide for classroom teachers* (3rd ed.). Boston: Allyn and Bacon.

Gold, M. (1980). *Did I say that?: Articles and commentary on the Try Another Way system.* Champaign, IL: Research Press.

Grigal, M., Dwyre, A., & Davis, H. (2006). *Transition service for students aged 18–21 with intellectual disabilities in college and community settings: Models and implications of success.* NCSET Publication. Retrieved January 19, 2007, from http://www.ncset.org/publications

Grossi, T.A., Banks, B., & Pinnyei, D. (2001). Facilitating job site training and supports: The evolving role of the job coach. In P. Wehman (Ed.), *Supported employment: Helping persons with disabilities go to work.* St. Augustine, FL: TRN Publications.

Grossi, T.A., Regan, J., & Regan, B. (1998). Consumer-driven training techniques. In P. Wehman & J. Kregel (Eds.), *More than a job* (pp. 119–148). Baltimore: Paul H. Brookes Publishing Co.

Halpern, A., Herr, C., Doren, B., & Wolf, N. (2000). *NEXT S.T.E.P.: Student transition and educational planning.* Austin, TX: PRO-ED.

Held, M., Thoma, C., & Thomas, K. (2004). "The John Jones Show": How one teacher facilitated self-determined transition planning for a young man with autism. *Focus on Autism and Other Developmental Disabilities, 19*(3), 177–188.

Holohan, A., & Costanbader, V. (2000). A comparison of developmental gains for preschool children with disabilities in inclusive and self-contained classrooms. *Topics in Early Childhood Special Education, 20*(4), 224–235.

Hughes, C., Copeland, S., Guth, C., Rung, L., Hwang, B., Kleeb, G., et al. (2001). General education students' perspectives on their involvement in a high school peer buddy program. *Education and Training in Mental Retardation and Developmental Disabilities, 36*(4), 343–356.

Individuals with Disabilities Education Act of 1990, PL 101-476, 20 U.S.C. §§ 1400 *et seq.*

Individuals with Disabilities Education Act Amendments of 1997, PL 105-17, 20 U.S.C. §§ 1400 *et seq.*

Individuals with Disabilities Education Improvement Act of 2004, PL 108-446, 20 U.S.C. §§ 1400 *et seq.*

Kohler, P. (2003). Transition-focused education: Foundation for the future. *Journal of Special Education, 37,* 174–183.

Kyeong Hwa, K., & Turnbull, A. (2004). Transition to adulthood for students with severe intellectual disabilities: Shifting toward person–family interdependent planning. *Research and Practice for Persons with Severe Disabilities, 29*(1), 53–57.

Kluth, P., Straut, D., & Biklen, D. (Eds.) (2003). *Access to academics for all students: Critical approaches to inclusive curriculum, instruction, and policy.* Mahwah, NJ: Erlbaum.

Lipsky, D.K., & Gartner, A. (1995, Spring). The evaluation of inclusive education programs. *National Center on Educational Restructuring and Inclusion Bulletin, 2,* 9.

Lipsky, D.K., & Gartner, A. (2006). Inclusion, school restructuring, and the remaking of American society. *Harvard Educational Review, 66*(4), 762–796.

Luecking, R., & Certo, N. (2002, December). Integrating service systems at the point of transition for youth with significant disabilities: A model that works. *NCSET Information Brief, 1*(4).

Luecking, R., & Fabian, E. (2000). Paid internships and employment success for youth in transition. *Career Development for Exceptional Individuals, 23*(2), 205–221.

Mank, D., Cioffi, A., & Yovanoff, P. (2000). Direct support in supported employment and its relation to job typicalness, coworker involvement, and employment outcomes. *Mental Retardation, 38*(6), 506–516.

Manset, G., & Semmel, M.I. (1997). Are inclusive programs for students with mild disabilities effective? A comparative review of model programs. *The Journal of Special Education, 31,* 155–180.

McDonnell, J., Hardman, M., Hightower, J., & Kiefer-O'Donnell, R. (1991). Variables associated with in-school and after school integration of secondary students with disabilities. *Education and Training in Mental Retardation, 26*(3), 243–257.

McDonnell, J., Thorson, N., Disher, S., Mathot-Buckner, C., Mendel, J., & Ray, L. (2003). The achievement of students with developmental disabilities and their peers without disabilities in inclusive settings: An exploratory study. *Education & Treatment of Children, 26*(3), 224–236.

Morningstar, M., & Torrez, J. (2003). Parents as systems change agents during transition. In D. Wandry & A. Pleet (Eds), *A practitioner's guide to involving families in secondary transition* (pp. 83–96). Arlington, VA: Council for Exceptional Children.

Mount, B. (2000). *Person-centered planning: Finding directions for change using Personal Futures Planning. A sourcebook of values, ideals, and methods to encourage person-centered development.* Amenia, NY: Capacity Works.

National Employer Leadership Council. (1996). *The employer participation model.* Washington, DC: Author.

National Transitional Longitudinal Study–2 (NLTS2). (2005). *Facts from NLTS2: High school completion by youth with disabilities.* Menlo Park, CA: SRI International. Retrieved December 8, 2006, from http://www.nlts2.org/pdfs/selfdeterm_factsheet_1122305.pdf

Neubert, D., Moon, S., & Grigal, M. (2002). Postsecondary education and transition services for students ages 18–21 with significant disabilities. *Exceptional Children, 34*(8), 1–11.

No Child Left Behind Act of 2001, PL 107-110, 115 Stat. 1425, 20 U.S.C. §§ 6301 *et seq.*

O'Brien, J. (1989). *What's worth working for? Leadership for better quality human services.* Syracuse, NY: Center on Human Policy.

O'Brien, J., & Lovett, H. (1992). *Finding a way toward everyday lives: The contribution of person-centered planning.* Harrisburg, PA: Pennsylvania Office of Mental Retardation.

O'Brien, J., & O'Brien, C.L. (1990). *A framework for accomplishment.* Decatur, GA: Responsive Systems Associates.

Pearpoint, J., O'Brien, J., & Forest, M. (1993). *PATH: A workbook for planning positive possible futures.* Toronto: Inclusion Press.

Phelps, L.A., & Hanley-Maxwell, C. (1997). School-to-work transitions for youth with disabilities: A review of outcomes and practices. *Review of Educational Research, 67*(2), 197–226.

Rehabilitation Act Amendments of 1986, PL 99-506, 29 U.S.C. §§ 701 et seq.

Rizzolo, M.C., Hemp, R., Braddock, D., & Pomeranz-Essley, A. (2004). *The state of the states in developmental disabilities: 2004.* Boulder: University of Colorado, Coleman Institute for Cognitive Disabilities and Department of Psychiatry.

Rogan, P., Banks, B., & Howard, M. (2001). Workplace supports in practice: As little as possible, as much as necessary. *Focus on Autism and Other Developmental Disabilities, 15* (1), 2–11.

Ryndak, D., Jackson, L., & Billingsley, F. (1999–2000). Defining school inclusion for students with moderate and severe disabilities: What do the experts say? *Exceptionality, 8*(2), 101–116.

Salend, S. J. (1999). The impact of inclusion on students with and without disabilities and their educators. *Remedial & Special Education, 20*(2), 114.

Sands, D., Kozleski, E., & French, N. (2000). *Inclusive education in the 21st century: A new introduction to special education.* Belmont, CA: Wadsworth Publishing.

School-to-Work Opportunities Act of 1994, PL 103-239, 20 U.S.C. §§ 6101 et seq.

Thoma, C., Baker, S., & Saddler, S. (2002). Self-determination in teacher education: A model to facilitate transition planning for students with disabilities. *Remedial and Special Education, 23*(2), 82–89.

Thoma, C., Rogan, P., & Baker, S. (2001). Student involvement in transition planning: Unheard voices. *Education and Training in Mental Retardation and Developmental Disabilities, 36*(1), 16–29.

Tomlinson, C.A., Stronge, J., & Cunningham-Eidson, C. (2003). *Differentiation in practice: A resource guide for differentiating curriculum.* Alexandria, VA: Association for Supervision and Curriculum Development.

U.S. Department of Labor. (1991). *What work requires of schools: A SCANS report for America 2000.* Washington, DC: Government Planning Office.

Villa, R., Thousand, J., Nevin, A., & Liston, A. (2005). Successful inclusive practices in middle and secondary schools. *American Secondary Education Journal, 33*(1), 33–50.

Wandry, D., & Pleet, A. (Eds.) (2003). *A practitioner's guide to involving families in secondary transition.* Arlington, VA: Council for Exceptional Children.

Wehman, P. (2006). *Life beyond the classroom: Transition strategies for young people with disabilities.* Baltimore: Paul H. Brookes Publishing Co.

Wehmeyer, M. (1996). Self-determination as an educational outcome: Why is it important to children, youth, and adults with disabilities? In D.J. Sands & M.L. Wehmeyer (Eds.), *Self-determination across the lifespan: Independence and choice for people with disabilities.* Baltimore: Paul H. Brookes Publishing.

Wehmeyer, M. (2001). Self-determination in transition. In P. Wehman (Ed.), *Life beyond the classroom: Transition strategies for young people with disabilities* (3rd ed., pp. 35–60). Baltimore: Paul H. Brookes Publishing Co.

Wehmeyer, M., Palmer, S., Agran, M., Mithaug, D., & Martin, J. (2000). Promoting causal agency: The Self-Determined Learning model of instruction. *Exceptional Children, 66*(4), 439–453.

Workforce Investment Act of 1998, PL 105-220, 29 U.S.C. § 794 et seq.

CHAPTER THREE

Toward Full Citizenship

New Directions in Employment for People with Significant Disabilities

PATRICIA ROGAN, MICHAEL CALLAHAN,
CARY GRIFFIN, AND DAVID HAMMIS

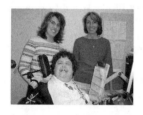

Supported employment, which took hold in the United States in the early 1980s, has been defined by the following features: paid employment in integrated work settings, for people with the most severe disabilities, with extensive, ongoing supports to get and keep employment. Since its inception, supported employment has expanded worldwide (Wehman, Revell, & Kregel, 1998) and has been used with people with all types of disabling conditions. After 25 years, hundreds of thousands of people previously deemed unemployable have secured integrated jobs (Mank, 1995; Wehman & Kregel, 1995), achieving better quality of life outcomes and personal satisfaction (Rogan et al., 2001). These demonstrations of success have proven that people with high support needs *can* work if the job is matched to their abilities and interests, and if they are provided the necessary supports. The impact of supported employment cannot be understated in the lives of individuals with high support needs. Earning a paycheck, gaining valuable work skills, interacting with co-workers, participating in the community, and contributing as taxpaying citizens have allowed individuals new options and opportunities as true consumers. Having a job and a paycheck is a powerful vehicle for changing other areas of one's life, including living, social, and leisure situations. In other words, employment is truly the anchor of a meaningful day and life.

CURRENT ISSUES AND BARRIERS

Unfortunately, supported employment, while initially conceptualized as a vehicle for systems change from segregated to integrated employment services, has not resulted in a large-scale shift in our service delivery system (Butterworth, Gilmore, Kiernan, & Schalock, 1999). If people with high support needs have proven their ability to work in real jobs in the community, then why would anyone need congregate, sheltered day programs anymore? Surely, funding agencies, family members, service providers, and people with disabilities would see the archaic and outdated service delivery system as broken, and demand a shift to integrated and individualized services! Not only has such a shift *not* occurred, but sheltered services have continued to grow in the United States (Braddock, Hemp, Parish, & Rizzolo, 2002).

There are many reasons for the current situation. Negative attitudes, insufficient funding; policies that support segregated services; lack of leadership; and low-skilled, low-wage, high-turnover staff issues are just some of the reasons. Ironically, rather than putting sheltered day services under intense scrutiny in terms of their costs, quality of services, and outcomes (or lack thereof), supported employment has been constantly under scrutiny and threat. For example, year after year the U.S. government threatens to remove earmarked funding for supported employment. Advocates throughout the country have had to fight constantly to maintain the gains that have been made.

One might view our current situation as a "best of times, worst of times" scenario. On one hand, supported employment continues to evolve, with exciting developments related to customization, self-employment, personal budgets, business leadership, innovative funding options, access to generic employment services, and technological advances. Some service provider organizations with strong leadership have undertaken the changeover process to close their facility-based services in favor of totally community-based services, as described in Chapter 8.

On the other hand, even the essential ingredients of supported employment, as listed above, are in jeopardy. People with high support needs continue to be excluded from supported employment, deemed unemployable, and relegated to day wasting programs or without any services. Ongoing supports are increasingly limited or nonexistent, as is funding for nonwork supports during the days. Supported employment, for some, has meant working with a group of people with disabilities with few, if any, co-workers without disabilities nearby. People may need to wait long periods of time for supported employment assistance, while they can often enter a sheltered facility immediately. Despite these threats and barriers, we must continue to focus on the essential elements of quality supported employment services, while promoting new innovations that offer true choice, control, individualization, and satisfaction for people with disabilities.

This chapter provides an overview of the essential components of quality supported employment services and describes recent innovative and effective practices that offer new directions and opportunities. Specifically, efforts to shift the system toward greater choice and control for people with disabilities are described. Customized employment and self-employment are discussed in depth, and other examples of innovative approaches for employment of people with high support needs are presented.

ESSENTIAL ELEMENTS OF SUPPORTED EMPLOYMENT

This section highlights essential elements and quality indicators of supported employment based on lessons learned during the past several decades. Supported Employment Quality Indicators (Rogan et al., 2001) were developed for the national APSE: The Network on Employment, an advocacy organization focused on supported employment.[1] The quality indicators are organized for individual job seekers, direct service practitioners, and organizational characteristics, but only the section for job seekers is included here. Next, typical steps in the employment process are briefly described.

APSE Quality Indicators for Individuals in Supported Employment—Individual Choice and Control of Resources and Supports

- Individuals explore career opportunities based on their interests, abilities, and needs via such experiences as vocational education classes, job shadowing, job try-outs, volunteer work, and actual employment.

- Individuals have ongoing opportunities to develop self-determination skills through active participation in information gathering, experiential learning, self-advocacy, and decision-making.

- Individuals direct their transition plan or employment plan to the maximum extent possible, with support as needed.

- Individuals control the resources, if desired, to purchase services and supports. Family members, personal advisors, and other trusted advocates assist individuals as needed.

- Individuals are assisted as needed to secure employment according to their individual desires, including the type of work environments, activities, hours, pay, supports, and so forth.

- Individuals participate maximally in interviews and in training and support procedures typical to workplaces.

- Individuals have necessary and appropriate accommodations, assistive technology, and individualized supports within and outside of their job.

- Individuals are connected to desired adult services, including generic supports, in order to pursue desired lifestyles.

---

[1]These quality indicators were developed by Patricia Rogan, Tammara Geary, and Dale Dileo with contributions from Renee Drouet, Dale Dutton, Karen Flippo, Tom Harrison, Brenda Harvey, Rob Hoffman, Pat Keul, Sue Killam, Debra Martin Luecking, Rebecca McDonald, and Bob Niemiec.

- Individuals pursue career advancement opportunities in order to develop skills, increase pay and responsibilities, or achieve other desired outcomes.
- Individuals develop satisfying relationships within and outside their job, as desired.
- Individuals are supported to participate in social activities within and outside their job, as desired.
- Individuals are compensated commensurate with others in the same position.
- Individuals have access to reliable, accessible, and affordable transportation.
- Individuals are assisted to manage their finances (e.g., banking, budgeting, benefits) as needed and desired.
- Individuals of retirement age are supported to pursue a variety of employment or postemployment options.

The Employment Process

An extensive body of literature exists about supported employment processes and strategies (e.g., Callahan & Garner, 1998; Hagner & DiLeo, 1993; Luecking, Fabian, & Tilson, 2004; Wehman, 2001). While there are many paths to obtaining and retaining a job, typical steps for securing wage employment are briefly outlined here. Strategies for self-employment are described in a later section.

Get to Know the Job Seeker   If a job seeker needs assistance to get and keep employment, the first essential step in the job search process is to get to know the individual well. Guiding questions include: Who is this person? What are their hopes and dreams, passions, strengths and interests, and support needs? What is the impact of their disability on daily life? What do they need to be successful? Who are the people closest to the individual who know him or her best? What type of role do they play and what support do they provide to the person? There are many ways to get to know a job seeker as a person, and the more natural the better. Rather than take the individual to a strange room with a strange person and ask them to perform strange tasks that may have no bearing on their job interests (i.e., typical of traditional vocational evaluation) (Rogan & Hagner, 1990), it is more appropriate and helpful to spend time with the person across familiar and unfamiliar people, settings, and activities. Obviously, the job seeker should be a primary source of information, as are the people who know the job seeker best. The process of getting to know the person, often called *discovery*, and the information that is gathered can be compiled in a personal profile (Callahan, 2004; Griffin, Hammis, & Geary, 2007).

Use Person-Centered Planning   As discussed in other chapters, person-centered planning is critical to the development of a roadmap for individualized services and supports. Many tools exist for person-centered planning (e.g., Making Action Plans [MAPs], Planning Alternative Tomorrows with Hope [PATH], personal futures planning, essential lifestyle planning) that assist people who know the job seeker best to plan with the focus person and take action for positive change. The planning process typically involves envisioning a desired future, identifying the hopes, dreams, interests, strengths, and support needs of the focus person, and developing a plan to achieve desired outcomes. Members of the planning team share responsibilities for actions and activities and reconvene periodically to check progress and make changes. Part of person-centered planning for employment should be targeting the type(s) of job the individual might like, characteristics or conditions of desired work environments and tasks, types of supports that might be needed, and identifying people who have connections to particular businesses. The information that is generated can be added to the personal profile and/or used to develop a portfolio to use during employer contacts.

As the concept of person-centered planning has spread to nearly every corner of the disability field, there are concerns that this powerful strategy has become a perfunctory requirement that must be performed once a year to meet funding requirements. Staff members have been heard to complain about the time required for such plans and families and individuals with disabilities have complained about the unfulfilled promises and the lack of input in the planning process. These criticisms have led some practitioners to shift control of person-centered plans from an agency/system perspective to one owned by the individual. Person-directed planning—a process that not only places the individuals as the center of planning concerns but also allows the person and family to direct the process—is emerging as a way to resolve problems associated with mundane person-centered plans.

Ensure Individualization Simply stated, individualization relates to the degree to which one's job is about the person or about factors outside the person—employers, systems, regulations, and so forth. In her testimony before the U.S. Senate, Secretary of Labor Elaine Chao (2001) described the concept of individualization quite elegantly: "As we invest in critical job training, we are giving workers the bargaining power they need to custom-design their jobs around their lives—instead of the other way around." This concept places the prospective applicant at the beginning of the job search (a "person-first" approach) instead of the more traditional "jobs-first" approach. This is a critical aspect of quality supported employment in that too often agencies and systems have turned to employers first, before looking closely at the needs, skills, and interests of the individual. By starting with the individual, it is possible to assure that supported employment is not just another jobs program. The list included next in this section explains what individualization and person-centeredness mean for supported employment.

- The job search begins with individual discovery of the applicant.
- Job development does not begin until *after* a plan has been developed.
- Person-centered employment planning meetings become the drivers of job development efforts instead of being cursory, required services.

- Job developers primarily represent one person at a time to employers.

- The factors of employment relating to the applicant are given priority over the presumed factors of employment relating to employers and the labor market.

- An applicant's best dimensions of performance are used to determine their contributions rather than their performance against others or against arbitrary standards.

Search for Possible Jobs that Would Be a Good Job Match   With the job seeker in mind, this step of the job development process involves canvassing area businesses to explore work settings and tasks that would match the job seeker's interests and abilities. Information about particular businesses can be gathered using a job analysis format. For example, business can be investigated in order to learn who is doing what, how, and for what pay? What is the nature of the work environment (e.g., physical layout and accessibility, characteristics of the workforce, potential for co-worker supports, employee dress, location in the community, transportation options)?

Learn About Employer Needs   If the workplace appears to offer a possible match with the job seeker, additional investigation into the business may be warranted. After all, employers appreciate knowing that someone has taken the time to learn about the nature of their business and their personnel needs prior to contacting them about hiring. Informational interviews, a tour of the business, and exploration of company literature are possible strategies for gathering helpful information.

Contact Employer(s) to Negotiate a Job   Employer contact typically involves discussing how the individual job seeker can meet employer needs, the support that can be provided to assist the employer, and negotiating specific features of a job, including tasks (beginning and future), work area, job training, accommodations, wages, benefits, hours, and other important conditions of employment. Obviously, this discussion is aimed at negotiating a "win-win" situation that meets the needs and interests of both the job seeker and employer. This is a key time to negotiate customized features of the job in order to meet the needs of the employer and employee.

Adhere to Natural Proportions   Although enclaves and work crews have been and continue to be viewed as part of supported employment, grouping people with disabilities in an immediate work area should be avoided. Grouping people with disabilities violates the natural proportion or distribution of people with disabilities that would be found in our community. Grouping tends to increase stigma, reinforce stereotypes, diminish opportunities for natural supports, ensure the presence of external paid support, and reduce the individualization of the person–job match.

Facilitate Natural Supports   In the past, job coaches assumed the primary role in training and supporting individuals with disabilities on the job. Yet workplace personnel know the job and the work culture best. It is very important for the employment specialist to stay out of the way and complement, rather than take over, training and support by designated supervisors or co-workers. If co-worker support does not occur naturally, the employment specialist can facilitate their involvement by helping them get to know the supported employee and assisting them to learn how to provide the type of support the individual needs. The employee with a disability should be central in identifying his or her support needs.

Facilitate Job Growth and Advancement   People with disabilities have often been placed in dead-end jobs with which they soon become bored. Depending on the needs and interests of the supported employee, opportunities should be developed for ongoing job growth and advancement, including horizontal (increasing the variety of tasks at the same difficulty level) and vertical (increasing the sophistication of the tasks) enhancement.

Monitor Job Satisfaction   It is very important to monitor the satisfaction of both the employer and the supported employee over time. Regular communication between the employer and the supported employee (and their employment specialist, if appropriate) is necessary to ensure that both parties are pleased with the situation.

The strategies above have been used to successfully assist individuals with high support needs in obtaining and keeping employment. Outcomes of supported employment vary from state to state and organization to organization. Most supported employees work part time (about 20 hours per week) and earn minimum wage. Many have entry-level, stereotypic (e.g., food service, janitorial) jobs. Many had little, if any, voice in their own job search. In response, some agencies began to embrace strategies that initiated and carried out the employment search not only from the *perspective* of the individual, but with the *direction* of the person with a disability. The groundwork was being laid for a new, more meaningful form of supported employment to emerge. This new version continues to value offering employment to *all* persons with disabilities who want to work, but it embraces a new set of values that are defining quality both within the disability field and in society as a whole.

Shifting Toward Choice, Control, Ownership, and Customization

Ever since Congress required that written rehabilitation plans be individualized within the Rehabilitation Act of 1973 (PL 93-112), we have been on a collision course with the offspring of individualization: choice, control, and customization. Table 3.1 illustrates the evolution of the factors influencing the disability field as a whole.

These factors, taken individually, may not seem to form a path of clear direction regarding changes that have influenced the direction of supported employment. However, when taken together, they form a picture of an

Table 3.1.   Timelines, catalysts, and changes in the disability field

Timelines	Catalysts	Changes in the disability field
1973	Rehabilitation Act	Individualized written rehabilitation plans
1975	Individuals with Disabilities Education Act (IDEA)	Individualized education programs
1980s	Integration in community and schools	Person-centered planning
1987	Part H of IDEA	Family control of resources
1990	Americans with Disabilities Act	Prohibits employer discrimination
1992	Rehabilitation Act Amendments of 1992	Informed choice in the rehabilitation process
1993	Retirement Savings Account Choice Demonstration	Choice, control of money, personal budgets
1994	Robert Wood Johnson Demonstration	Home of Your Own Project, home-ownership
1995	Robert Wood Johnson Demonstration	National self-determination projects
1998	Workforce Investment Act	Individual training accounts, choice
2001	U.S. Department of Labor	Customized employment projects

inevitable evolution of services. We can see the journey of our recent past and also plot out the clear mandates of the future of supported employment. Whenever services are about the individual, the individual will want input, the right of refusal, and will ultimately demand choices and control of the process.

CHOICE AND CONTROL OF SERVICES AND RESOURCES

One confusing factor that often sets employment apart from other aspects of human services involves the relationship between people and the jobs that they have. Generic labor policy in the United States has focused far more on macroscopic issues such as job growth and economic development than on individual factors such as interest, goodness-of-fit between an individual and their job, and personal passion. Indeed, most citizens seem to find their way to careers more by serendipity than by design. Therefore, it is little wonder that those who assist individuals with disabilities to become employed have, at times, utilized those same generic, often arbitrary, approaches within supported employment. In other words, they may see supported employment as more of a general jobs program than as a set of strategies designed to offer an individualized, working lifestyle to people who might not otherwise work.

However, this general approach to employment is at odds with two powerful factors: disability policy and the needs of people with significant disabilities. Beyond its necessity as a fundamental concept for employment, individualization is a catalyst that generates other, more powerful concepts: choice, control, ownership, and customization. The following section will examine each of these factors and their impact on supported employment.

Choice

Choice in supported employment can be thought of in terms of options and prerogative. "Is there an array of current and potential services and outcomes for me to choose from?" and "Do I get to decide what might work best for me?" are essential questions of choice-driven services. The history of disability services for people with significant disabilities placed a caring professional in charge of selecting the right services and outcomes for the individual. The concept of choice requires that we shift that authority to those whom we support. The first clear indication that choice was to become a component of supported employment was in the Rehabilitation Act Amendments of 1992 (PL 102-569). Congress directed vocational rehabilitation services to assure the provision of "informed choice" and to assist persons with disabilities to become

> Full partners in the vocational rehabilitation process, making meaningful and informed choices…in the selection of employment outcomes for individuals, services needed to achieve the outcomes, entities providing such services and the methods used to secure such services. (Rehabilitation Act Amendments of 1992)

In other words, people with disabilities are to have both choice and prerogative within this powerful federal legislation. The list on this page describes what choice means for supported employment.

- Individuals must be allowed to choose their providers of service from among an array of current and potential service providers.

- Individuals must be assisted to understand the complexity of the decisions and possible alternatives through the use of independent advisors, paid or volunteer, who work for the person, not the system.

- Individuals must choose desired outcomes, the services needed to achieve those outcomes, and the methods used within the services, with assistance as necessary.

- Individuals have primary say throughout the discovery, planning, development, and support process and are consulted on all decisions that affect their lives.

- Families and other nonpaid supporters, chosen by the individual, have a critical role in offering assistance.

- The role of professionals shifts from the traditional prerogatives regarding authority to make decisions to that of a partner who shares in the decision making.

- In addition to selecting providers and outcomes, individuals also decide the pacing of services, the level of personal investment, as well as the relevance of outcomes selected.

Control

Control is to choice as person-directedness is to person-centeredness. In other words, control ups the service ante in favor of the individual yet again. In 1993, the Rehabilitation Services Administration was directed by Congress to fund large-scale national demonstration projects designed to examine the role of informed choice within the rehabilitation process. Seven projects were funded for a 5-year period, each with a different view of the role and scope of choice. By the end of the demonstration in 1998, six of the seven projects had embraced strategies that allowed individuals not only to exercise *choice* of the sort described above, but they had also established methods that allowed participants to *control* the public resources available for their rehabilitation (Callahan, 2000).

The control of public resources by the user of those resources is yet another example of the extension of individualization. It is virtually inevitable that as people have more and more choices, they will also want to control as many aspects of service as possible. This is not to say that control of resources implies that public funds are simply handed over to the individual with a disability in a sort of "pay and pray" strategy that they will achieve their outcomes. Rather, response to the value of offering individuals increased control of resources has resulted in a dizzying array of options that allow for individuals to direct the expenditure of funds in pursuit of employment outcomes—personal budgets, individual development accounts, cash-out plans, vouchers, micro-boards, self-directed support corporations, and Plan to Achieve Self-Support (PASS) plans. And, to facilitate and support fiscal control strategies, there are now services that did not previously exist—brokers, fiscal agents, leasing agents, advisors, benefit specialists, and plan consultants.

Strategies to offer fiscal control to individuals vary along a continuum that ranges from placing funds directly in an account controlled by the person to an individual component within an agency's larger budget. Regardless of the option utilized, these strategies must offer, at a minimum, the following assurances.

- The funds are dedicated to the individual and relate to specific outcomes and associated costs in the person's employment plan.

- Funds cannot be paid out, removed, or used alternatively without approval of the individual.

- Sensible fiscal control strategies are included that assure the outcomes/ costs targeted in the plan are consistent with outcomes obtained and prices paid for outcomes.

- The individual has full access to information about the account.

Figure 3.1 provides examples of various options for fiscal control from the least restrictive to more restrictive. Regardless of the strategy used, fiscal control strategies all offer the opportunity for the user of services to direct the manner in which the funds will be spent. There are, of course, strings attached. It is

Degree of restriction	Strategy for fiscal control
Less restrictive	*Cash payments directly to the individual*
↓	*Direct deposit into a dedicated service account (i.e., cash-outs)*
↓	*Dedicated vouchers for certain services*
↓	*Individual Development Accounts (i.e., shared saving accounts)*
↓	*Plan to Achieve Self-Support plans from Social Security Administration*
↓	*Micro-boards/self-directed support corporations*
↓	*Individual accounts/personal budgets held by third party*
↓	*Dedicated case accounts held by system (e.g., vocational rehabilitation, developmental disabilities)*
More restrictive	*Individual service line item within an agency's larger budget*

Figure 3.1.   Degree of restriction and strategy for fiscal control.

imperative to assure that the concepts of individual control of resources and fiscal integrity are fully compatible within choice-driven services.

The list in this section explains what control means for supported employment.

- All parties—individuals, families, providers, system personnel, and bureaucrats—have to respond to the demands of new learning and behaviors required by choice and control.

- Service providers must begin to trust individuals, families, and other nonpaid entities and to welcome them into full partnership and participation.

- It is necessary to accept that a handoff must occur between staff and individuals of both the authority and responsibility of directing public funds. If the handoff is done well, a true partnership can emerge based on trust and shared interest.

- Providers and system personnel have to practice giving up power in every interaction with individuals with disabilities and their families.

- School transition programs for students with disabilities must begin to include experiences that will enable students to participate, as much as possible, in controlling resources for employment.

- Personnel must strive to remove barriers to control within all levels of the disability field.

Ownership

The term *ownership* is used here to describe the degree to which the individual with a disability "owns" the job or small business they engage in for their employment. Historically in the disability field, human service agencies have acted as proxies between employees with disabilities and their employers. For example, when setting up enclaves and work crews, agencies have negotiated a relationship with employers on behalf of employees with disabilities. In these cases, the employment relationship is actually between the supported employee and the human service agency, not with the employer. The employer maintains a contract relationship with the agency, pays the agency, and holds the agency responsible for the expectations stated in the contract agreement.

There are many problems with this agency-controlled practice. How much control does an employee truly have if the agency owns the employment relationship? Can a job genuinely be individualized if there is a question as to whose job it is? Beyond the contradictions implied in these questions, proxy relationships pose a number of problems for people with disabilities. When the employment relationship is between the agency and the employer, the employee becomes interchangeable, depending on the employer's demands and concerns. Employees with more significant impact of disability, such as behavioral challenges or low productivity, are often replaced with individuals with fewer or more manageable challenges. The proxy relationship affects employer attitudes also. Instead of committing to the applicant with a disability, the commitment is to the agency, as long as the job demands are met.

Similar concerns exist regarding small business development. As sheltered workshops faced the pressure to change their focus from contract work to community employment (Murphy & Rogan, 1995), some developed small businesses to employ individuals once served in the facility. These businesses were characterized by issues related far more to the agency and the local market economy than to certain individuals with disabilities. In other words, the businesses were developed first, then individuals were selected to work there. While this concept was undoubtedly an improvement over segregated, contract work in a sheltered workshop, it is a far cry from individual ownership of a microbusiness that is derived from a consideration of the person's skills, needs, and passions in relation to the needs of a local economy. In order for supported employment to be relevant in the current times, it is imperative that the employment relationship or the small business, as appropriate, be owned by the person with a disability, not the human service agency. Below is a list describing what ownership means for supported employment.

- The employment relationship in a supported employment job should be between the employer and the employee, not with the human service agency.

- When the employment relationship is between the employer and the supported employee, there is a greater opportunity for naturalness, for a deeper commitment by the employer, and for a rationale to resolve workplace issues rather than replacing the employee with a substitute worker.

- Ownership of the job by the supported employee indicates that human service agencies no longer intend to insert themselves as proxies with employers and that genuine supported employment belongs to the individual, not the agency.

- Small business development should be individualized to the skills, needs, and interests of specific persons with disabilities and the businesses should be owned by the individual, not the agency.

Customization

Since the earliest days of supported employment, it was recognized that some individuals, possibly many, would need an individually negotiated relationship with employers in order to become successfully employed (Nisbet & Callahan, 1987). After all, if one accepts that disability exerts a real and significant life impact on people who have been characterized as having severe disabilities, it follows that such people are likely to struggle in their effort to compete with so-called typical applicants for arbitrary job descriptions in the competitive workplace. This awareness led practitioners who were committed to employment of people with significant disabilities to include an additional dimension to the existing components of supported employment—negotiation of an individualized job description (Callahan, 1990, 2000; Hagner & Dileo, 1993).

The essence of individualized supported employment was that the essential responsibilities of the job (Americans with Disabilities Act of 1990 [PL 101-336]) were negotiated on behalf of the applicant in a manner that met the needs of the employer and the unique contributions of the applicant. This approach allowed access to employment for people with even the most significant disabilities, as long as a willing employer needed the contributions of the supported employee and the necessary supports and accommodation were available. As the concept of individualized supported employment matured through the 1990s, the more generically-acceptable term of *job restructuring* was adopted by many practitioners. The shift to job restructuring allowed employers, applicants, and professionals in the broader employment arena to understand a concept that many thought was, at best, a niche strategy, and at worst, an example of quasi-employment. However, the term job restructuring was used to indicate similar, but different, strategies. A more descriptive and universally acceptable term was needed.

In 2001, the Office of Disability Employment Policy (ODEP) of the U.S. Department of Labor issued a solicitation for grant activity for local workforce boards, mandated by the Workforce Investment Act of 1998 (PL 105-220) to compete for funding related to a demonstration of a newly coined concept of employment known as *customized employment*. ODEP defined customized employment in the following manner:

> Customized employment means individualizing the employment relationship between employees and employers in ways that meet the needs of both. It is based on an individualized determination of the strengths, needs, and interests of the person with a disability, and is also designed to meet the specific needs of the employer. It may include employment developed through job carving, self-employment or entrepreneurial initiatives, or other job development or restructuring strategies that result in job responsibilities being customized and individually negotiated to fit the needs of individuals with a disability. Customized employment assumes the provision of reasonable accommodations and supports necessary for the individual to perform the functions of a job that is individually negotiated and developed. (ODEP Customized Employment Grants Notice, 2002)

This definition provides both clarity and acceptance concerning the strategy of negotiating individualized job descriptions and employer relationships on behalf of applicants with disabilities. Beyond that, the definition of customized employment provides legitimacy for a concept often thought not to represent "real" or quasi-employment. The concept of supported employment, as it did with the individualized strategies developed in the 1990s, benefits from this definition in that it encompasses all the values and aspects of supported employment—supports, individualization, choice, control, ownership—*and* it is relevant in the broader employment arena. This aspect is critical in that supported employment, without customized employment, has been viewed as appropriate only for people with significant disabilities. By embracing customization, supported employment aligns with mainstream employment strategies effective for anyone who has a complex life and needs the flexibility of customized employment to become successfully employed.

As in supported employment, negotiations to customize employment relationships target two facets of a job in relation to meeting employer needs: 1) the specific job duties to be performed by the applicant and 2) the general conditions of the job and work situation, such as hours of work, times of work, location within a workplace, supervisory and support relationships, and so forth. Specific duties of customized jobs may be divided into four distinct categories of job descriptions.

- *Carved jobs*: Job descriptions based on tasks derived from a single traditional job

- *Negotiated jobs*: Job descriptions based on tasks derived from a variety of jobs

- *Created jobs*: Job descriptions based on heretofore unmet needs of an employment setting

- *Microenterprises*: Customized employment duties based on a very small business, owned by the individual, that meets unmet needs of a local market or economy

The general conditions held by an employer for a given job may also be negotiated to meet the needs and preferences of the applicant. Supported employment has traditionally embraced this concept in terms of work hours and other aspects relating to general expectations that might be open to negotiation—supervisory relationships, flex time to deal with uncertain mental health issues, location within the workplace to perform one's duties, ideal times of the day to work, and other similar factors. The key ingredient is voluntary negotiation with employers to meet legitimate workplace needs.

While critical distinctions among these various types of customized jobs have yet to be fully determined, it is fair to say that even if these categories do not currently represent the typical way in which employers and/or customers interact with employees, supported employment practices in the past decade have established the legitimacy of such strategies.

The list that follows describes what customization means for supported employment.

- By embracing customized employment, supported employment is enhanced by the inclusion of generic, business-friendly concepts that allow anyone who wants to work to do so.

- The applicant must drive the job search, not existing employer relationships, labor market needs, or agency connections.

- By assimilating customized employment within supported employment, the opportunity exists to broaden the definition of supported employment to include others in the generic community, to anyone with a complex life.

THE SELF-EMPLOYMENT OPTION

Ryan is 21 years old. He owns and operates Ryan's Artworks in rural Montana. Three years ago, he was destined to a life in the local segregated day activity center. Ryan, like so many individuals with multiple significant disabilities leaving high school, had virtually no choice in the matter. It was the day activity center or nothing. Fearing this for their son, Ryan's parents pulled together a team of people from the Rural Institute at the University of Montana and came up with a plan. Ryan, who loves art, would start his own business, with management and sales assistance coming from his family. Family support is a common element in successful small business (U.S. Department of Commerce, 2000).

The business design involved Ryan using a sponge dipped in watercolors and dabbing or swirling it on a blank canvas. The result is a colorful background that was then purchased by a local well-known artist who used these backgrounds for still life and landscape works of art. Ryan made other products as well, with the assistance of his family and day program staff. While Ryan is not getting rich, not yet anyway, he is earning money, contributing to his family's income, and planning for life in the community. Thinking creatively resulted in a unique business model, raised the expectations of all involved, and short-circuited an almost certain future of inactivity and poverty.

WHY SELF-EMPLOYMENT?

As stated in this chapter, more individuals with significant disabilities enter day programs than enter the world of work. Stemming this tide takes the hard work and vision exemplified by Ryan, the local provider agency, his family, and others. While self-employment appears to be a complex undertaking for anyone with a significant disability, it is a rather basic concept and the foundation of community life. Long before there was wage employment, there was self-employment. Thomas Jefferson's agrarian vision of the yeoman farmer and Horatio Alger's poor-boy-makes-good scenarios are both examples of this country's rich heritage of self-sufficiency and of individual accomplishment. This cultural phenomenon should not be denied to individuals with disabilities any more than the dream of owning a home and starting a family to able bodied individuals who do not experience disabilities.

Indeed, in the United States, self-employment for people without disabilities is flourishing. Over 20 million Americans now work in home-based businesses and the self-employment rate is growing at over 20% annually. Between 1990 and 1994, microenterprise (businesses employing from 1 to 5 workers) generated 43% of all the new jobs in the United States, and in the past decade, 60% of microenterprises were owned by women and created more jobs than the entire Fortune 500 combined. Furthermore, despite folklore to the contrary, small business succeeds at a rate approaching 80% (Access to Credit, 1998; Forrester, 1996; Sirolli, 1999; U.S. Department of Commerce, 2000). With the unemployment rate slowly rising to a current figure of over 5% nationally, loyalty to companies continues to fade, creating an even more fertile environment for small business exploration and growth. People with disabilities are being swept up in this worldwide movement after years of chronic unemployment.

Why self-employment? The answer is obvious: We know where past efforts have taken us. Individuals with significant disabilities have a high unemployment rate, are infrequently engaged in their communities, have few close personal friends or intimate relationships, but generate millions of dollars in services-related capital, and are surrounded by professional staff. What could be the harm in trying a new and different strategy for a change?

Does self-employment make sense for someone who has little or no verbal communication, rocks in his seat most of the day in a work activity center, appears unmotivated, occasionally strikes out violently, and does not appear to value money or a day's work? Typically, all these behaviors, or lack of behaviors, are the result of long-term isolation, coercion, and boredom. The description of the individual reflects a "deficit frame of reference" that leads many to assume that the individual is unsuited for employment. Self-employment is grounded in the belief that all people have strengths, interests, preferences, and an innate ability to perform work competently when offered choices, respect, support, and opportunities. Abandoning stereotypes and taking a "strengths-based" approach is a proven process (Callahan & Garner, 1998; Griffin & Hammis, 1996, 2001).

Examples of Self-Employment

A middle-aged gentleman who spent most of his life in institutions, workshops, and group homes was brought to the attention of Rural Institute staff in Montana. From the strengths-based perspective, he had many positive attributes: a pleasant smile, an interesting sense of humor, and a manner that made those around him feel at ease. Two noteworthy interests or strengths included his collection of stuffed animals in his group home bedroom, and the enjoyment of his volunteer work at the local nature center where wounded wild animals are rehabilitated prior to releasing them back into the wild. At the nature center, he fed and groomed the animals, interacted with other staff and volunteers (although he is largely nonverbal), and helped out with other light chores.

Unfortunately, this gentleman was considered too disabled to work by agency personnel, and even though the nature center valued him as a volunteer, they did not have the revenue for or the interest in hiring him. A proposal was developed to sell stuffed animals at the center with assistance from the provider agency staff who would manage his books and inventory, and called upon the nature center staff to help with daily operations such as money exchanges. The design of the business was not typical, and management of the business was different from most, but sales flourished and a strong partnership grew as the entrepreneur paid 10% of profits to the nature center for rent and minor assistance with the largely self-serve operation. Six years later, the business has expanded to sales of stuffed animals in three down-town stores, with inventory and sales being managed by each store. The stuffed ani-mal business owner is now seen as a regular on Main Street and is viewed as a success by the local developmental disability provider, which helped him move into his first apartment. And, because he has a bank account in the company's name, he has amassed over $8,000 in cash, well above the $2,000 limit for someone receiving SSI payments.

By taking a strengths-based approach, deficits melted away and attributes rose to the front. A little creative support, costing far less than the day program, along with a good business design, led to success.

In another case, Jerome, a young man with autism, was constantly running from the sheltered workshop in rural North Carolina. Using a person-centered approach to employment development, it was discovered that in his family, Jerome was known for his light touch when transplanting seedlings and for his love of big trucks and farm equipment. In fact, his running from the workshop always occurred when big trucks or farm equipment drove by; Jerome was simply trying to catch a ride.

A job development plan sought to find Jerome agricultural wage employment. As often happens however, a chance meeting with brothers who owned a local farm, and the random donation of a greenhouse to the provider agency, led to the establishment of Jerome's Greenhouse next to the brother's roadside produce stand. After several licensing delays, Jerome's Greenhouse opened its doors, supplying specialty plants and vegetables through the roadside stand and starting seedlings for the brother's farm. Jerome was once considered unemployable due to the severity of his disability and his unpredictable behavior. Today, he has an employment specialist who helps with production, and rich natural supports from his family and the two brothers who own the farm and teach him the trade, and who also give him occasional rides on tractors! The business will gross over $20,000 in its first year, and inspired over a dozen agency staff to discuss their own personal small business ideas with several of the authors. Jerome's success transformed others by serving as a role model for self-employment.

In the two examples above, self-employment evolved as a natural option once a vocational profile was developed that pointed out likes, dislikes, pre-

ferred environments, supports needed and available, and existing and potential resources. Self-employment is only one option, and not always the best one.
The decision to start a business must be based on the individual's dreams and
desires, the ability to create or respond to market needs, and the availability of
supports. Of course, the need for business supports is often used to discourage
people with disabilities from pursuing self-employment.

Business Partnerships   Small business supports typically involve
assistance with production or service delivery (operations), business planning,
sales and marketing, and bookkeeping or accounting. Of course, these are
common supports required for any business. As service dollars become more
flexible and portable, *personal* control of resources will become more widely
accepted and this will lead to easier arrangement of business supports. For
now, creative leveraging of supports may be necessary. For instance, in Ryan's
case, his support came from an exclusive deal with the artist to create canvases.
By developing an informal partnership, Ryan generated revenue immediately,
built his skills and reputation, and has been able, with family and agency
support, to expand products. Ryan still relies on sales of greeting cards,
featuring his backgrounds and the artist's foreground paintings, for his
primary revenue.

At the nature center, a business-within-a-business model worked best.
This provided a steady stream of customers drawn past the stuffed animals
and utilized existing employees to casually help out with the daily business
operations. Disability agency staff helped with the books and inventory.

Jerome's greenhouse is another business-within-a-business that utilized
disability agency support for production and bookkeeping, while also creating
a symbiotic relationship with the farmers who train to their specifications in
order to guarantee they are getting the best possible goods to sell in their roadside stand. Jerome's success is integral to the farm's success. Jerome, through
his small business, has become a vital and contributing force in the local economic development movement and not someone seen only as a taxpayer burden or passive member of the community.

Self-employment for people with significant disabilities makes sense for
several reasons. First, self-employment is a growing and substantial form of
employment in our market economy. It makes sense for people with disabilities to try their hands at a fast growing employment sector. Also, it allows flexibility with hours, what tasks are performed, and so forth.

Second, self-employment offers the only substantial option available
under our Social Security and Medicaid/Medicare systems to accumulate personal wealth and manage income in a way that is predictable and controllable.
Under Medicaid and SSI regulations, an individual beneficiary cannot accumulate more than $2,000 in cash resources, unless the cash resources are shel-
tered in a restricted irrevocable trust managed by someone else, or in a Plan to
Achieve Self-Support (PASS). A PASS is a powerful and useful employment
tool, but it is restricted to employment-related spending only and cannot be
used for any other purpose, such as buying a house.

A small business owner receiving SSI, Medicaid, or Medicare can have unlimited funds in a small business checking account for legitimate operating expenses as defined by the IRS and SSA under rules identifying Property Essential for Self-Support. A business owner can accumulate operating cash and other business capital and have substantial net worth in the business and can then sell the business and use the money to purchase a home. Self-employment creates the opportunity for increasing wealth and personal equity without penalty. Wage employment offers no such opportunity.

Third, self-employment makes sense for people with significant disabilities because Social Security benefits provide a financial cushion—income for survival—during the business start-up phase and often through the life of the entire business. The cash flow analysis for any business must include a breakeven analysis: the point when the business generates enough income to cover expenses. For a small business owner without a disability, who has no other source of income, the business must break even and provide survival income as well. Substantial cash resources may be needed early in the business simply to pay daily living expenses. However, as noted above, most people with disabilities have Social Security benefits to cover daily living expenses, so the business is not required to generate survival income; it simply has to reach the breakeven point.

Vocational rehabilitation and other employment services can access Small Business Development Centers (SBDCs) and the Small Business Administration (SBA) for help with business plans. It is important to note that developing cash flow analysis and profit analysis requires knowledge of Social Security and Medicaid/Medicare regulations, which typical SBDCs and SBA advisors do not have. For instance, if someone started selling gourmet dog biscuits, the following scenario might occur. If the fixed cost to sell the biscuits is $100 per month and the cost per order of biscuits sold (e.g., cost of ingredients, amortized equipment, rent) is 50% of the selling price, and the selling price per order of biscuits is $8.00, then the breakeven point per year is $2,400 in sales, or 300 orders. Profit analysis would show that if $6,000 in biscuits were sold (750 orders per year), then the profit for that year would be $1,800 or $150 per month. However, if the person is on SSI, which is reduced $1.00 for every $2.00 earned after the first $85, then the SSI monthly check will be reduced by $32.50 per month or $390 per year. This $390 can be projected and SSI will reduce the SSI check each month based on the projections, or it can be paid back to SSI as an overpayment at the end of the year when the business taxes are filed. If it is projected, SSI reduces the check, and if cash flow is unbalanced due to seasonal sales, then the business owner could end up with some months where he or she is not able to meet living expenses. The discretionary net personal profits are reduced from $150 per month to $117.50 per month due to the interaction of the SSI system rules.

SBA and SBDC staff generally do not understand these rules and regulations and require assistance in factoring in the interactions of SSI and Social Security Disability Income checks from Social Security. SSI does not balance net self-employment income on a month-by-month basis but by law has to divide the entire year by 12 in order to perform its reduction calculations. This is a significant benefit to self-employment that is not available in wage employment and allows for large fluctuations in income that do not impact benefits or Medicaid monthly. Another significant advantage to SSI rules and self-employment is the fact that if the business is exceeding projections to SSI and the owner chooses to reinvest the excess profit back into the business, the "reduction" interactions with SSI can be controlled, thus avoiding an SSI over-payment while simultaneously growing the business. This is not an option with wage employment, in which SSI reductions cannot be managed or avoided.

Fourth, self-employed people with disabilities may have access to alter-nate sources of capital to build their business. Conventional small business loans and investors for business start-ups are difficult and expensive for peo-ple without disabilities to acquire. Banks prefer not to make small business loans unless substantial resources are leveraged as collateral, and even then prefer not to be involved in small business launches, but rather choose to wait until the business is established and profitable. To access loans, the business and business plan often have to be well-developed and show high growth potential. Individual investors are the exception rather than the rule. Often only business ideas and applications that show high growth potential for buy-outs or "harvesting" receive revenue from such sources. Venture capitalists look for companies that will grow dramatically, and only 2% to 3% of all pro-posals are successfully funded and venture capitalists rarely invest in small firms.

People with disabilities can access a variety of capital sources, such as state vocational rehabilitation, Social Security PASS plans (Shelley, Hammis, & Katz, 2001), and "Intensive Services" under the Workforce Investment Act. Of course, family funds are also a traditional source of financing, and as agencies expand the use of personal budgets, more business starts are sure to come.

Fifth, self-employment works because it can be a good fit with the individual. Traditionally, self-employment is seen as being beyond the capabil-ities of people with significant disabilities. Understanding the person in his or her home, local community, and day-to-day context of living reveals oppor-tunities for self-employment. Self-employment can be used to match the small business owner's preferences, gifts, and unique contributions to a money-making operation when no wage employment options are readily available. Self-employment allows for the creation of a finely matched work opportunity designed specifically for someone that does not fit the standard employee molds while respecting context and natural supports for a unique, profitable, and viable form of community employment.

DESIGNING A SMALL BUSINESS

There are many examples of business plans available on the Internet and from the local SBDC. SBDCs are located in most population centers and are typically found in the white pages of the phone book. They can also be located by call-ing the local Office of Economic Development, usually located in the blue pages of the phone book, or by contacting the chamber of commerce. SBDCs do not normally write business plans but instead offer constructive assistance on them and provide valuable information on local markets. They also offer classes on business development that, while they may not be academically appropriate for owners with significant disabilities, do provide a networking opportunity and educational value to support staff and family members. While most successful businesses in the United States do not have a formal plan, one is recommended in order to think constructively about the future, to plan for cash flow, to critically analyze competition and customers, and to prove to various funding agencies that the individual is indeed serious about the business.

CONCLUSION

Employment is the natural state for adults in Western society. Whether individuals choose wage employment or a version of self-employment, it should be a core element of adult lives. Although self-employment is certainly not the most desirable option for everyone, its availability expands the likelihood of moving past segregation.

This chapter has provided an overview of key elements of successful supported and self-employment options, and examples of their implementation. Employment supports must always begin with the person and seek jobs, products, and services fitting their talents and circumstances. Matching personal profiles with market demand has the potential to connect people with the most significant disabilities to their community through continual commercial and social interaction with co-workers and customers.

REFERENCES

Access to Credit. (1998). *Small enterprise, big dreams* [Videotape]. Frederick, MD: Access to Credit Media Project.

Americans with Disabilities Act of 1990, PL 101-336, 42 U.S.C. §§ 12101 *et seq.*

Braddock, D., Hemp, R., Parish, S. & Rizzolo, M. (2002). *The State of the States in developmental disabilities: 2002 study summaries.* Boulder, CO: University of Colorado, Coleman Institute for Cognitive Disabilities and Department of Psychiatry.

Butterworth, J., Gilmore, D., Kiernan, W., Schalock, R. (1999). *State trends in employment services for people with developmental disabilities.* Boston: Institute for Community Inclusion.

Callahan, M. (1990). *Final report of the National Demonstration Project on Supported Employment.* Washington, DC: United Cerebral Palsy Association.

Callahan, M. (2000). *The meaning of choice: Implications for systems and providers.* Report for the Presidential Task Force on Employment of Adults with Disabilities.

Callahan, M., & Garner, B. (1998). *Keys to the workplace: Skills and supports for people with disabilities.* Baltimore: Paul H. Brookes Publishing Co.

Forrester, A. (1996). Beyond job placement: The self-employment boom. In N. Arnold (Ed.), *Self-employment in vocational rehabilitation: Building on lessons from rural America.* Missoula, MT: RTC Rural Rehabilitation.

Griffin, C.C., & Hammis, D. (1996). *Street wise guide to person-centered career planning.* Denver, CO: CTAT.

Griffin, C.C., & Hammis, D. (2001). Self employment as the logical descendant of supported employment. In P. Wehman (Ed.), *Supported employment in business.* St Augustine, FL: Training Resource Network, Inc.

Griffin, C., Hammis, D., & Geary, T. (2007). *The job developer's handbook.* Baltimore: Paul H. Brookes Publishing Co.

Hagner, D., & Dileo, D. (1993). *Working together: Workplace culture, supported employment, and persons with disabilities.* Cambridge, MA: Brookline Books.

Luecking, R., Fabian, E., & Tilson, G. (2004). *Working relationships: Creating career opportunities for job seekers with disabilities through employer partnerships.* Baltimore: Paul H. Brookes Publishing Co.

Mank, D. (1995). The underachievement of supported employment: A call for reinvestment. *Journal of Disability Policy Studies, 5*(2), 1–24.

Murphy, S., & Rogan, P. (1995). *Closing the shop: Conversion from sheltered to integrated work.* Baltimore: Paul H. Brookes Publishing Co.

Nisbet, J., & Callahan, M. (1987). *The vocational strategy.* Gauter, MS: Marc Gold & Associates.

Novak, J., Rogan, P., Mank, D. & DiLeo, D. (2003). Supported employment and systems change: Findings from a national survey of state vocational rehabilitation agencies. *Journal of Vocational Rehabilitation, 17*(1), 47–57.

Office of Disability and Employment Policy Customized Employment Grants Notice, 67 Fed. Reg. 43154–43169 (June 26, 2002) (to be codified at 29 C.F.R. pt. 95).

Rehabilitation Act of 1973, PL 93-112, 29 U.S.C. §§ 701 *et seq.*

Rehabilitation Act Amendments of 1992, PL 102-569, 29 U.S.C. §§ 701 *et seq.*

Rogan, P., & Hagner, D. (1990). Vocational evaluation in supported employment. *Journal of Rehabilitation, 56,* 45–51.

Rogan, P., Grossi, T., Mank, D., Haynes, D., Thomas, F., & Majd, C. (2001). *Changes in wages, hour, benefit, and integration outcomes of former sheltered workshop participants who are in supported employment.* Report for the President's Task Force on the Employment of Adults with Disabilities. Indiana University: Institute on Disability and Community.

Shelley, R., Hammis, D., & Katz, M. (2001). *It doesn't take a rocket scientist to understand and use Social Security work incentives* (5th ed.). Missoula, MT: Rural Institute/University of Montana.

Sirolli, E. (1999). *Ripples from the Zambezi.* Gabriola Island, British Columbia: New Society Publishers.

U.S. Department of Commerce. (2000). *Report on small business success.* Retrieved December 20, 2000, from http://www.usdoc.gov

Wehman, P. (Ed.). (2001). *Supported employment in business: Expanding the capacity of workers with disabilities.* St. Augustine, FL: Training Resource Network, Inc.

Wehman, P., & Kregel, J. (1995). Supported employment: At the crossroads. *Journal of the Association for Persons with Severe Handicaps, 20*(4), 286–299.

Wehman, P., Revell, W.G., & Kregel, J. (1998). Supported employment: A decade of rapid growth and impact. *American Rehabilitation, 24*(1), 31–43.

Workforce Investment Act of 1998, PL 105-220, 29 U.S.C. §§ 794 *et seq.*

CHAPTER FOUR

Creating Inclusive Postsecondary Educational Environments

VALERIE SMITH AND PAMELA M. WALKER

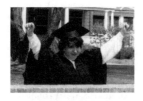

Increasing numbers of people with disabilities are enrolling in postsecondary education (Blackorby & Wagner, 1996; Getzel & Wehman, 2005), and increasing numbers of colleges and universities are making efforts to provide accommodations and supports for students with disabilities (Getzel & Wehman, 2005; Pierangelo & Crane, 1997). At the same time, this enrollment is still approximately 40% below that of the general population (Stodden, 2005). In a 1999 report of a longitudinal study of students with and without disabilities, The Center for Educational Statistics found that, of a group of students who completed high school by 1994,

> Students with disabilities were much less likely to be even minimally qualified for admission to a 4-year college than were students without disabilities…Thus, even though a majority of students with disabilities aspired to a college degree, less than half were at least minimally qualified…This suggests that students with disabilities may not be getting the academic preparation necessary for them to achieve their goals. (U.S. Department of Education, 1999, pp. 31–32)

Included among these students with disabilities enrolled in postsecondary education are a small but growing number of students with cognitive impairments (see, e.g., Hamill, 2003). Research has found that people with disabilities, including those with cognitive impairments, benefit from postsecondary education, with lower rates of workshop use and higher rates of competitive employment following postsecondary education experiences (Gilmore, Schuster, Timmons & Butterworth, 2000; Gilmore, Schuster, Zafft, & Hart, 2001). However, until recently, very few people thought of postsecondary education as an option for those with cognitive or severe developmental disabilities.

In the past, when adults with developmental disabilities wanted to continue their education beyond high school years, the only options were segregated classes (i.e., to learn basic academics and skills). For example, during the
1970s, programs such as College for Living emerged, a special program on college campuses offering courses for adults with developmental disabilities
(Neubert, Moon, Grigal, & Redd, 2001).

During the 1980s and 1990s, there was a significant expansion of college-
based programs. Some of these programs were focused specifically on students
transitioning from high school and were established in conjunction with local
school districts (e.g., Grigal, Neubert, & Moon, 2001). There is great variation
among these programs, with some that operate primarily as separate programs, offering special courses and some inclusion in regular college classes,
and others that focus on supporting students to participate in regular college
classes and other aspects of campus life. Two of the pioneering programs
include the OnCampus program associated with the University of Alberta,
Canada (Developmental Disabilities Bulletin, 1994; Developmental Disabilities
Bulletin, 1997; Frank & Uditsky, 1988), established in 1987, and the ENHANCE
program at Trinity College in Vermont (Doyle, 1997), established in 1989. Both
the OnCampus program and the ENHANCE program were designed not as
special programs but to provide "equal access to college resources and equal
opportunities for involvement in campus and community activities for people
with developmental disabilities" (Doyle, 1997, p. 16). Key characteristics of
these programs include individually determined supports for students and
ongoing discussion of career goals and interests. As described by Doyle (1997),
there were two core values underpinning the inclusion of adults with disabilities at Trinity College.

- The college values the preparation of students who will treasure diversity
  among people and who will base their valuation of others on a respect for
  the inherent worth of the human person.

- The college values itself as a place that calls each of its members to be
  accountable for her/his gifts and to use them in ways that serve the community and work toward the betterment of society.

Since the mid-1990s through the present time, there has been continued development of initiatives on campuses to provide inclusive learning experiences
for individuals with disabilities, including those with cognitive disabilities. In
addition, during this same time period (from the mid-1990s to the present), an
increasing number of individuals are gaining access to postsecondary education opportunities through their own initiative, and with the assistance of family members, support staff, and service agencies. In order to do so, individuals
who are past school-age are drawing on a variety of sources of support. For
example, some are eligible for support through the developmental disabilities
service system (e.g., through the Medicaid waiver or other sources) to assist
them with their pursuit of postsecondary education. In addition, the vocational
rehabilitation system may be a source of financial and other types of support
for postsecondary education and related expenses, while people who receive
Supplementary Security Income (SSI) are eligible for certain postsecondary

education supports (Golden & Jones, 2002; Luecking & Murphy, 2000; Seybert, 2002).

This chapter gives some examples of means by which people with developmental disabilities are gaining access to and participating in postsecondary education. This includes students who are auditing courses and taking courses for credit, as part of universities, community colleges, and adult/continuing education programs.

Chapter 2 describes the role that on-campus programs play in transition to meaningful lives in the community. This chapter focuses, in part, on a more in-depth description of one on-campus program and profiles of a few of the students who have participated in this program. This is followed by a section that offers some examples of students who have gained access to postsecondary education in a variety of other ways. The chapter concludes with a discussion of key issues that need to be addressed in order to promote increased opportunities for access to postsecondary education for all.

THE ONCAMPUS PROGRAM AT SYRACUSE UNIVERSITY

The OnCampus program at Syracuse University facilitates the inclusion of a small number of Syracuse City School District students in university classes and vocational and social experiences. OnCampus is based on a program at Asbury College in Kentucky called College Connection (Hall, Kleinert, & Kearns, 2000) that supports several transition-age students with moderate to severe disabilities in college experiences. Like College Connection, OnCampus includes young adults with moderate to severe disabilities in daily campus-based experiences. Unlike College Connection, OnCampus students spend all of their instructional day at Syracuse University and in the surrounding community.

The idea of OnCampus was brought to the district special education director by the Vargo family, whose oldest daughter, Ro, has Rett syndrome. With a copy of an article about the Asbury College program, the Vargos approached Ed Erwin, the Syracuse City School special education director, and Doug Biklen, a Syracuse University professor prominent in the field of inclusive education. Planning began in the spring of 2000, and OnCampus invited its first seven students to participate during the fall of 2000.

OnCampus exists as a partnership between the city school district and Syracuse University's School of Education. Under this agreement, Syracuse City Schools provides transportation for its students, an inclusion facilitator who coordinates student educational programs and supervises school staff, and six educational technicians who provide direct support to OnCampus students. In addition, the school district is legally responsible for the safety of students while at the university. Syracuse University provides access to university classes and activities (each student has a student identification card that gives them access to the same locations and activities that matriculated university students have access to), and a program coordinator who serves as liaison between OnCampus students and staff and Syracuse University. This coordinator also supervises university undergraduates who spend 2 hours per week during the semester with OnCampus partners through several service learning courses offered by the School of Education. OnCampus has a planning board, comprised of OnCampus staff, the city school special education director, the Syracuse University faculty sponsor, parents, and various adult service agency representatives. This board meets regularly to review OnCampus progress and to brainstorm for the future. At its initial planning meetings, the OnCampus board decided that the project would target students who otherwise would be very unlikely to gain access to postsecondary education, especially students with more severe disabilities.

CASE EXAMPLES

Ro had been included in regular classes with support throughout her education. She expressed a desire to go to college and her parents wanted to assist her in exploring this possibility. Based on this, they initiated discussions about developing the OnCampus program, and once this program was established, Ro became one of the first participants. Ro was strongly interested in social justice issues, and she chose courses related to that interest, such as Introduction to Sociology. Due to her Rett syndrome, Ro did not speak; instead, she pointed to words, indicated "yes" and "no" by nodding or shaking her head, and occasionally used a simple augmentative communication device that has overlays and prerecorded messages. Ro had some trouble with physical mobility and needed time to move between classes and activities. She had a reputation for being careful about opening up to new people but was very social once she got to know her student partner.

Sam, another OnCampus student, came with labels of moderate mental retardation and a communication disorder. He usually used one-to-three-word phrases to communicate, or asked a nearby teaching assistant to answer questions for him. His reading level was not clear. While his school records indicated that he read at about a first-grade level, many university students noted that he seemed to easily navigate the Internet and occasionally asked questions about things that he could have known only if he had been reading text. Sam got a DynaMyte communication device during his time with OnCampus and was learning to use it, although he usually preferred to rely on his other methods of getting meaning across. Sam was a warm, friendly guy known for his concern for the health and happiness of his fellow students and his insistence on having pizza and soda with lots of ice for lunch every day. Sam took courses focusing on health and nutrition.

Jon, a student with Down syndrome, is a talented musician who plays piano, violin, and clarinet and also has his black belt in tae kwon do. Jon had fairly good verbal and reading skills, although he had trouble answering questions that ask for specific details or names. He was studying for his driver's permit exam at the time of his involvement in OnCampus, and was working on developing his public speaking skills. At the university, he took a course on the music industry and one on public speaking. Jon enjoyed being with college-age peers but sometimes seemed shy with new people or in large groups.

OnCampus offers its students educational experiences that are similar to those of their university peers. OnCampus students who are considering continuing postsecondary education have the opportunity to experience many aspects of university student life. By auditing classes, students are able to practice being in an environment that may have different demands than high school. Students have the opportunity to explore interests and develop competencies through taking university classes. For example, as described previously, one of Jon's future goals is to perform music and tell audiences his story. Thus, the courses on public speaking and on the music industry were directly related to his interests and goals. OnCampus students gain an understanding of the pace and demands of postsecondary education while having the flexibility of not having to meet all the course requirements. With the guidance of the city school staff, OnCampus students learn about adaptations that work for them in academic settings, and they learn to see themselves as competent learners.

In addition to the support for class participation, OnCampus students are provided support for experiencing college life more broadly. The partnerships with the university students give OnCampus students the chance to learn about daily life on a college campus from the perspective of their same-age peers. They see their university student partners budget their time and money, learn their way around campus (and where to find the best pizza among the variety of places to eat, on and off campus), and experience ways that typical college students socialize with each other.

In conclusion, campus programs, particularly those that offer support for inclusion in the campus community, can be an important means of offering access to postsecondary education and the experience of college life for students with cognitive disabilities. In addition to such campus programs, there are a variety of other ways that individuals with developmental disabilities are gaining access to postsecondary education opportunities.

PURSUIT OF POSTSECONDARY EDUCATION ON AN INDIVIDUALIZED BASIS

Among the increasing numbers of students with developmental disabilities who are gaining access to postsecondary education opportunities are those who have worked out these arrangements on an individual basis (Weir, 2001). Some people have worked out these arrangements on their own, with the assistance and support of family or friends. In other cases, special initiatives, such as the Robert Wood Johnson Foundation's state self-determination projects (Bradley et al., 2001), have helped create opportunities that had not previously been available. For instance, in Vermont, Michelle was a young woman who was interested in attending college. Team members from the Vermont Self-Determination Project helped her figure out how to use her Medicaid waiver funding to support her college participation (e.g., Walker, Harris, Hall, Smith, & Shoultz, 2000). Finally, local agencies and state service systems that provide employment and community living services are increasingly assisting people with other meaningful and relevant daytime pursuits, including postsecondary education opportunities. For example, in their efforts to respond more fully to the individual needs and desires of people they support, staff at Common Ground, in Littleton, New Hampshire, have gained competency in the resources and steps necessary to assist people with going to college. Following are some brief case examples of some individuals who have pursued postsecondary education.

Molly studied early childhood education at a community college, earning a teaching assistant certification in May 2003. She has done extensive national public speaking about her life and her advocacy. In past schooling, because of her label of Down syndrome, Molly was placed in segregated classrooms. Molly described the background of her desire to go to college:

> Even though I was in a segregated class, I did have dreams. I always wanted to go to college. I knew exactly who I wanted to be when I was in ninth grade because I did an internship with a teacher that I knew, and she inspired me. So, I said, I want to go to college, like my brother and sisters.

After high school, Molly took a 2-year course in early childhood education at the county Board of Cooperative Educational Services, a public entity that provides educational programs and services to school districts in New York State. After this, she had to take a test prior to admission to the community college. Upon admission to the college, Molly and her parents arranged with school administrators that she would spend 4 years working on her associate's degree. Molly knew of this college because it is a popular one with students from her small, rural town.

The college had a learning center that assisted students with special needs. One of the staff members at the learning center arranged for Molly to have tutors for certain subjects. When Molly first enrolled in the college, she and her parents met with the director of the learning center to discuss some of the most effective ways that tutors could support Molly. This information was helpful for the director in selecting and orienting tutors for Molly. Some of the ways they assisted her included reviewing class notes and other materials with her. Also, when there was a quiz or test, the tutors read the questions to Molly. Overall, Molly felt very positive about the support she received from the learning center. At the same time, she felt that, as the first student with Down syndrome, she helped educate people at the learning center about supporting people with developmental disabilities.

In addition to the support from the learning center, Molly received 16 hours a week of support from a young woman named Beth, paid for through her Medicaid waiver. Much of Beth's support focused on schoolwork, although in addition, she and Molly spent some time hanging out or doing fun things in the community. For instance, Molly enjoys horseback riding, so they did this together.

Beth attended classes with Molly and helped her with taking notes. Outside of class, Beth devised a variety of strategies for helping Molly learn the material. She did this with input from Molly, Molly's family, colleagues at her workplace, and the professors. Beth explained, "I've learned to become very good friends with the professors, and they help me."

Overall, one of the keys to this opportunity for Molly was being part of her individualized education program (IEP) meetings. "When I was in high school, I was fortunate that I could go to my IEP meetings," Molly said. "Some students are not allowed to go to theirs. For me, I was fortunate that I could go and decide what I needed to achieve my goals for what I wanted to learn. And I want other students to have that same opportunity."

For Molly, some of the most positive aspects about going to college were the support she received and the ability to pursue her career. While most of her professors "have been wonderful," one of the challenges was the small number of faculty who did not seem supportive. Also, Molly's mother expressed that a difficulty, both in high school and college, was gaining access to a social life.

In the future, Molly would like to work in early childhood education. Also, she wants to continue with public speaking, educating people about disability issues. As Molly put it, "Telling them my experiences; helping people to understand more about people with disabilities, so there's less discrimination. There's so many people out there that don't know, and they get so afraid. I don't want them to be afraid; I want them to welcome people."

Joanne has been using facilitated communication (FC) for 12 years. In the fall of 1989, when she was in middle school, Joanne's speech therapist began working with her to learn FC. The following spring she wrote her first sentence. She began mainstream classes and went to all general education classes the following fall. Joanne is now majoring in psychology at a small liberal arts college. To participate in classes and complete coursework, Joanne, who is labeled autistic, uses FC. Prior to admission, Joanne went for an interview at the college. She feels that college administrators reacted positively to her desire to go to college: "I think that the people at college believed that I could do the work, and I pretty much was welcomed to the college community."

With funds from the New York State Office of Vocational and Educational Services for Individuals with Disabilities, Joanne hires other students to facilitate with her in class. She has obtained them mostly through notices on college bulletin boards. While she has been successful in finding people to facilitate with her, they have not always done this well. Joanne becomes frustrated because she wants to be able to find good facilitators.

Most of Joanne's facilitators are full-time students, so they have limited availability. Thus, while they assist her in class, her mother has assisted her with most of her work beyond the classroom, such as writing papers. Joanne says sometimes it is hard having to rely so much on her.

Joanne's mother also describes the hard work that it takes from Joanne and herself. She feels in some ways as though Joanne is doing a lot more work than she would be if she was not a student with a disability. It has also been more work than initially *anticipated for Joanne's mother, who commented, "I've had a couple of students work on papers with her, but mostly I've done that myself, which I didn't really realize I was getting into." However, while there has been a lot of work, Joanne's mother also talks about the positive aspects of this work together. "All the stuff she's learned has been a wonderful education, so it's been a blessing in disguise."*

Overall, Joanne is very pleased to be in college. She says, "I want to get a college degree because I think that the degree will mean the way to a successful future." In the future, she would like to work for the FC institute. In her schooling and pursuit of her career, she hopes to be a role model for others who would like to have similar opportunities.

Robert,[1] who has a visual impairment and seizure disorder, was 38 years old at the time he enrolled in an adult education course titled "Effective Speaking and Human Relations." He initially enrolled because he thought it might assist him with a telephone sales job. Soon thereafter, he lost the job but continued the course for the next 3 months. Instead of increasing his sales potential, the class offered Robert a chance to meet people and to become a member of a community, for a limited period, with others who shared the experience. This course took place every Wednesday night for 14 weeks, from 6:30 p.m. to 10 p.m. The course cost $850, which was paid through Robert's Supplemental Security Income (SSI) Plan to Achieve Self-Support (PASS). SSI PASS plans arise out of an SSI regulation that allows SSI recipients to set aside funds, which would otherwise be considered as available to meet their needs, to be committed to a plan to achieve self-support, resulting in eligibility for SSI.

The classes generally consist of about 30–40 students, a class instructor, and 5–8 graduate assistants. These graduate assistants are former students who have returned to help teach the course as well as to assist students in whatever way is needed. This support occurs both during class time and beyond it, and the type of support is determined by the needs of the particular student.

There were a number of aspects of the philosophy and design of the course that were key to Robert's full participation. The philosophy into which all students are indoctrinated mandates support of others in the group. When the course instructor announced that Robert was taking taxicabs to and from class, two men immediately volunteered to give him rides. The availability of supports for all students, based on need, facilitates provision of assistance for participants with disabilities. The graduate assistant who supported Robert was willing to adapt the level of support he typically gave students to Robert's special needs. Finally, the general emphasis on cooperation and teamwork created an atmosphere where Robert not only felt a sense of accomplishment, but also of connection. As Robert put it,

---

[1]From Fisher, E. S. (1995). A temporary place to belong: Inclusion in a public speaking and personal relations course. In S.J. Taylor, R.Bogdan, & Z.M. Lutfiyya (Eds.), *The variety of community experience.* Baltimore: Paul H. Brookes Publishing Co; adapted by permission.

I have gotten a lot out of this class. I have gained a lot of self-confidence. At the beginning, I was really afraid to get up and talk in front of all of you. Now, it's not so hard...I have also met a lot of great people in this course, and I think that we have all learned a lot together. (Fisher, 1995, p. 128)

TOWARD INCLUSIVE POSTSECONDARY EDUCATION OPPORTUNITIES FOR ALL

This section addresses steps that need to be taken in order to create further opportunities for all individuals to pursue postsecondary education. These steps are grouped in three categories: preparing for college, individualized support for college participation, and the role of colleges and universities.

Preparing for College

Many of the individuals featured in this chapter spent at least part of their school years in segregated classrooms, yet they dreamed of attending college and are now doing so without having had the benefit of exposure to the general curriculum. Jenn is a young woman with autism who majored in psychology at a private college in central New York (Fox, 2003). She wryly describes her precollege school experiences as doing

> Interesting things like sequencing beads and making toast...I am going to college without benefit of a real education...I began at Penn State by auditing one class. The next semester I took two courses for credit. By the fourth semester I applied as a provisional student, and I was accepted as a matriculated student by the fifth semester. It was difficult as a college student because I did not have a formal high school background like my peers. (Seybert, 2002)

With each reauthorization of the Individuals with Disabilities Education Act (IDEA), it becomes increasingly clear that the intent of the law is to provide supplementary aids and services that give students maximum access to the general curriculum for elementary and secondary school years. Measurable annual goals and short-term objectives, in the language of the law, are intended to relate to meeting the child's needs to enable the child "to be involved in and progress in the general curriculum" (IDEA 2004 [PL 108-446], Sec. 614). Ideally, then, students who receive support under IDEA should have IEPs that provide them with access to the same curriculum as their peers. It follows that this access would be best attained in the regular classroom, and, again, this appears to be the intent of IDEA, as special education is designed to ensure that the child "be educated and participate with other children with disabilities and nondisabled children" (IDEA 2004, Sec. 614).

Students who have been included in regular classrooms throughout their school careers are more prepared for postsecondary education in a number of ways, including having a broader academic base from which to understand new course material, understanding classroom norms and expectations, and being better prepared to meet admission requirements of postsecondary institutions.

Many of the students featured in this chapter dared to dream about attending postsecondary education despite the fact that they were not given access to ideal educational preparation or support to help make the dream a reality. If school personnel (i.e., teachers, school psychologists, guidance counselors, and others in positions of influence) considered each student, disabled or not, as "potential college material" from the earliest grades, perhaps all students, disabled or not, would be better prepared to enter postsecondary education upon graduation. Students with disabilities would graduate with useful diplomas that carry Carnegie units (i.e., secondary school units representing one year of work in a particular subject) rather than IEP diplomas, and would have access to the same guidance counselors, college fairs, and other helpful resources as their college-bound peers. Transition plans would be built around exploring different kinds of postsecondary educational options rather than limiting students to the traditional food service, custodial, and retail (i.e., stocking shelves) vocational experiences that fill past (and many current) transition plans. Based on her research with teachers, Smith (1997) emphasizes both the importance of teacher expectations for full participation as well as scheduling and support strategies to promote full participation.

Schools can help students with disabilities be better prepared for postsecondary education by helping them understand their disability and the ways it impacts them on an individual basis, as well as the ways to identify accommodations and technology that best support their learning characteristics. The student who has help learning to recognize what strategies will help her or him gain more from class, rather than just accepting what the special educator provides, is more prepared to ask for needed accommodations at the postsecondary level. For example, Jon, one of the OnCampus students who was profiled previously, has difficulty judging how much time has passed, although he can tell time with his watch. One of Jon's morning tasks was to make a list of the things he needed to accomplish during the day, prioritize this list, and decide how much time to devote to each task. As the year progressed, he was able to use this list and manage his time more independently, rather than relying on others to tell him what to do. Clearly, this is a skill that each of us must learn to be successful adults, and Jon learned strategies to help with his difficulty monitoring time.

One major difference between IDEA 2004 and Section 504 of the Rehabilitation Act of 1973 (PL 93-112) is in how support services are accessed. Once a student under IDEA has been identified as having a disability, she or he is entitled to ongoing support services and is assigned to a special educator whose responsibility is to monitor the student's progress. Once the student leaves high school, however, she or he must request services and take ownership of her or his progress; there is no IEP team out there whose job is monitoring the student's progress, or suggesting different accommodations if those currently being provided do not work (Johnson, Sharpe, & Stodden, 2000). Individualized transition planning teams can help with transition by ensuring that students have the opportunity to learn necessary skills and helping to arrange for needed ongoing supports. However, in order to be best prepared for this transition when they are in school, it is important that students be involved in the development and monitoring of their own IEP. In addition, special education teachers who support their students to take an increasingly active role in this process as the student nears graduation help students be better prepared to weather the change in support styles between high school and postsecondary education.

Related to the need for schools to support students in understanding their disability is the need for schools and other entities to help students learn to advocate effectively for their needs (Johnson et al., 2000; Preece, 1995; Yuen & Shaughnessy, n.d.). Special education programs, and countless IEP goals, reflect the concept of student independence, particularly in reference to discrete tasks. If these same programs considered the ability to effectively ask for help (i.e., promoted self-advocacy) as a skill linked to independence, students could spend their school years learning ways to get the help they need to succeed in their lives after high school.

Individualized Support

In order for students with cognitive and developmental disabilities to be included in postsecondary education, there is need for support to be determined based upon the individual needs of the student. Many universities have disability support services offices, which may be of assistance (see further discussion later in this chapter). However, often students with more significant disabilities will require supports that go beyond the extent that such offices are able to provide. This might include hiring a support person as well as acquiring specific equipment. It is sometimes very challenging to arrange all the necessary supports and funding sources for those supports. For instance, the college may provide some supports, the developmental disabilities service system may pay for others, and the vocational rehabilitation system may pay for others (Luecking & Murphy, 2000; Seybert, 2002). Seybert noted that even students with strong advocacy skills may find it challenging to pull together all the pieces. In order to arrange these, there is need for collaboration between the individual and others, including family members, transition personnel, college personnel, service coordinators from the developmental disabilities service system, and representatives from the vocational rehabilitation system.

Based upon the experience of many of the students described previously in this chapter, it is crucial to have a support person assisting both during class time and with the coursework associated with the class (e.g., readings, papers, studying for tests). The structure of the OnCampus program provided that assistance to participants. Other students used family members or support staff hired with funds from the service system (e.g., individuals with developmental disability labels are eligible for funding from the developmental disabilities service system, such as a Medicaid waiver, and/or from the vocational rehabilitation system). Based upon the experience of students with support staff, there are some important lessons about these support staff and their role.

First, support staff must have a concept of the students they support as being competent learners. In part, this concept is intuitive (e.g., believing that all people are capable and can learn); in part it needs to be promoted through university-based training and service agency staff training. Once this concept is a reality in the support person's mind, they are more able to provide the kinds of support (e.g., note taking, adapting materials or instruction) that give the student responsibility for learning.

In addition, having support staff who are familiar with and comfortable in academic settings can be helpful, particularly those who have had some post-secondary experience themselves, and possibly even in the area of interest of the student. In order to help students master the class material, the teaching assistants or support staff must be fairly independent, be competent note tak-ers, and must themselves keep up with the course readings and activities. Those who have not had such experience might have difficulty thinking of strategies to assist the students they support in learning the required material and completing the required coursework. For example, it was discovered that some of the OnCampus teaching assistants, eager to ensure that their students were successful in class, were completing assignments *for* their students rather than *with* them. Having the student copy work composed by the assistant, rather than composing and typing their own answers, didn't provide the stu-dent with a real learning experience. Not only did the students need to think of themselves as competent learners, so did teaching assistants!

For others, however, especially those who had their own postsecondary experiences, supporting students and suggesting innovative ways of adapting course materials came more easily. Their comfort in the college classroom, and in working with course content, helped the students they supported have more confidence and success in class. Sam, one of the OnCampus students, had a teaching assistant who helped him develop and program a presentation for his Health and Safety class onto his communication device. For Sam, who had always been in segregated classes where he was not expected to give presenta-tions in front of a group of people, this was a very new experience. His pride in his work helped Sam overcome his usual shyness in front of unfamiliar peers, and the presentation was a success.

Support staff may benefit from training that helps them expand and increase their skills. For example, the OnCampus program offered support to teaching assistants to help them develop skills adapting course materials, with positive results. As teaching assistants have success adapting materials, they also developed confidence and began to recognize the potential in the students they supported.

Finally, there is need for support for students to be part of the college community. College is more than just a place to take classes; it is a community, with perhaps smaller subcommunities within it, where students feel varying degrees of belonging. Some students with disabilities report feeling excluded from the social life of the campus. There is recognition of this, and the intent of programs such as OnCampus and ENHANCE is to provide support for broad-based participation in college life.

The Role of Postsecondary Institutions in Student Success

The previous section offered suggestions to help students with disabilities be prepared for postsecondary education as they leave the IDEA umbrella. In this section, we outline ways in which postsecondary institutions can be better prepared to accept and support all students. There has been some recent attention in the field regarding strategies to improve the quality of higher education for students with disabilities (Ben-Moshe, Cory, Feldbaum, & Sagendorf, 2005; Getzel & Wehman, 2005; Izzo, Hertzfeld, Simmons-Reed, & Aaron, 2001). For example, "Postsecondary Education: A Choice for Everyone," is a project funded by the Office of Special Education and Rehabilitative Services at the Institute on Disability at the University of New Hampshire. In part, it will focus on providing statewide training and professional development for faculty and staff of colleges regarding inclusion of students with disabilities. And, there has been some attention to the issue of providing a quality accommodated experience, or going beyond compliance with the Americans with Disabilities Act and other laws and regulations (Beyond Compliance Coordinating Committee, n.d.; Jones, 2002). There are an increasing number of colleges that are making concerted efforts to become fully accessible to all students (Battle, 2004; Bergin & Zafft, 2000), and there are an increasing number of resources around the country to assist colleges in this, including demonstration projects funded by the U.S. Department of Education, Office of Postsecondary Education, as well as national resource centers such as the Center on Postsecondary Education and Disability at the University of Connecticut.

Students with disabilities bring a particular kind of diversity to campuses that are already welcoming increasing numbers of students from diverse cultural, religious, or ethnic backgrounds, as well as students with a variety of sexual orientations. Just as exposure to students with a variety of personal histories and practices expands the possibilities for learning and understanding for all students, so do students whose learning characteristics, appearance, or behavior differ from the mainstream. By welcoming students with disabilities through flexible interpretations of admissions policies, full-time status, and support, postsecondary institutions broaden the opportunities for other students to develop acceptance of human variation in all its forms.

The campus community benefits in a number of ways from having students with disabilities in its classes, libraries, gyms, and social spaces. Beyond the curb cuts and automatic door openers that many people without disabilities use, the variety of adaptations used by students with disabilities have potential benefits for classmates without disabilities. Graphic organizers, outlines, and visual charts used by students with learning disabilities can help all students follow presentations of complicated information. Students who use sign language interpreters in class discussions require that classmates take turns when speaking, which helps everyone in class hear and be heard by others. Closed-captioning on videos may help those who have trouble processing auditory information, or to whom English is a less-familiar language. Finally, adaptations that make the campus accessible to students with disabilities also make students with disabilities accessible to the campus community. Like those from other countries, nondominant cultures, and nondominant races, students with disabilities may have different life experiences that challenge others to think about the world from a perspective beyond their own, and that challenge understandings of society, societal values, and social justice.

Postsecondary institutions can create opportunities to provide the campus community with more direct exposure to disability-related understanding by including disability in diversity-related programming, or by inviting prominent speakers with disabilities to campus, just as they invite prominent speakers from other populations to address the campus population. For example, people like John Hockenberry, who uses a wheelchair as a result of a spinal cord injury, and Adrienne Ashe, who is blind, speak on topics broader than just their status as individuals with disabilities. Hockenberry's experiences as a journalist take him to the sites of conflicts around the world, and Ashe is a well-known feminist scholar.

As disability types broaden, this is challenging universities to provide adaptations and accommodations that are more diverse (Johnson et al., 2000; L'Institut Roeher Institute, 1996). Most students with disabilities who attended college in the past had vision, hearing, mobility, or learning disabilities. While these student are attending college in increasing numbers, so are students like Jenn, Molly, and Ro, who present more diverse communication and learning styles. At the same time, students with disabilities make up a large number of those dropping out (Izzo et al., 2001; U.S. Department of Education, 1999). We propose that there are many things that can be done on an institutional level that will improve access to postsecondary education for all students, not just those with disabilities. Students whose learning style requires something other than the old lecture-and-test format found in many postsecondary classrooms challenge instructors to think creatively about how they impart understanding. For example, most university instructors, while willing to include an OnCampus student in their class (in fact, many are intrigued by the idea), have a particular manner of delivering instruction in their class that does not best suit the needs of the students with intellectual disabilities. Postsecondary institutions can provide faculty and course instructors with training in universal instruction, which incorporates strategies to teach students with a wide variety of learning styles (i.e., through small group work; formats that incorporate visual, auditory, and hands-on experiences; or through activities that synthesize theory and practical application) (Battle, 2004; Scott, McGuire, & Shaw, 2003). Each of us has a particular style of receiving and working with information that suits us; if instructors are supported to learn new ways to teach course concepts, all students will have a better chance of understanding those concepts. Classrooms will become a more interesting place for every student. Most campuses have resources already available to them that can help design training that helps instructors improve their teaching; for example, schools of education or other teacher training programs have faculty members whose expertise is in the area of pedagogy.

Offices of disability services at the postsecondary level are a critical resource. Yet, they do not seek out students with disabilities in order to offer them accommodations; the student must ask for what is needed. Often, the student also must negotiate what kinds and frequency of support they need. Most offices of disability services at the postsecondary level have a lot of background in supporting students with visual, auditory, or mobility impairments, or with learning disabilities, as these are the categories of students with disabilities who most frequently attended college in the past (U.S. Department of Education, 1999). Disability services offices may have much less familiarity with developmental disabilities like Down syndrome, autism, or Rett syndrome. As mentioned earlier, students with an increasing variety of disability labels are now attending postsecondary institutions. Offices of disability services that have traditionally supported students with a limited variety of disabilities may need help learning to accommodate the needs of students whose disabilities have not yet been encountered on campus (Hamill, 2003). Institutions can support those working in these offices to seek professional development opportunities and encourage them to work in collaboration with departments on and off campus that might have expertise or ideas about supporting students who have these more diverse disability labels. Offices of disability services must also be strongly encouraged to work more collaboratively with students to understand the unique learning styles and accommodations they need. Some disability services offices are beginning to form student advisory boards that can provide them with ongoing information and support, which is a very promising practice.

CONCLUSION

The inclusion of students with disabilities in postsecondary education environments has many sorts of benefits for the students with disabilities. In addition, inclusion offers many benefits to the postsecondary education community. These benefits include:

1. *Having students with a range of disabilities adds to the diversity at the university.* This helps broaden the definition of diversity from the traditional boundaries of ethnicity, religion, and sexual orientation, providing opportunities to learn the value of many kinds of diversity.

2. *Participation of students with disabilities within the campus community provides opportunities for that community to question old ideas about who belongs in higher education.* Students with disabilities show that, given adequate support, they are successful students, friends, and members of the university community. Students with disabilities allow others to examine ideas about social justice and the meaning of disability labels in society.

3. *Having students with diverse abilities and disabilities helps break down stereotypes about competency, communication, interaction, and relationships.* Having students with diverse abilities and disabilities in a campus community helps others develop skills conversing with people who don't speak, or who com-

municate in unique ways. This helps in learning how to develop relationships with people who seem quite different from us. This helps us learn that there are many important ways that we are all the same.

4. *Students with disabilities spur faculty to think differently about how, and whom, they teach.* OnCampus students bring the class a variety of adaptations that demonstrate innovative ways to teach all students. These students make unique contributions that add to the richness of the course for all students. They demonstrate to faculty that learning and intelligence are expressed in many ways.

In the not too recent past, postsecondary education for students with cognitive disabilities was rarely a consideration. In recent years, this mindset has shifted and opportunities have increased. At the same time, these opportunities are still limited and there is need for increased efforts in this area (Getzel, Flippo, Wittig, & Russell, 1997). In order for such inclusion to be successful, first, there is need for belief in the competency of students with disabilities. Second, there is need for supports based on the needs of individual students. And, third, there is need for collaboration to provide the necessary supports (National Council on Disability, 2003). This may entail collaboration from individuals, families, school systems, vocational rehabilitation, service coordinators, and adult support agencies (e.g., vocational services, residential services). Across the country, there are emerging some examples of initiatives aimed at fostering such collaboration (see, e.g., Hart, Zimbrich, & Ghiloni, 2001). With these elements in place, there will exist many varied opportunities for all students to participate in postsecondary education.

REFERENCES

Americans with Disabilities Act of 1990, PL 99-435, 42 U.S.C. §§ 12101 *et seq.*

Battle, D. (2004). Project Success: Assuring college students with disabilities a quality higher education. *The ASHA Leader, 6,* 14–15.

Ben-Moshe, L., Cory, R.C., Feldbaum, M., & Sagendorf, K. (Eds.). (2005). *Building pedagogical curb cuts: Incorporating disability in the university classroom and curriculum.* Syracuse, NY: Syracuse University.

Bergin, M., & Zafft, C. (2000). Creating full access for all: Quinsigamond Community College. *Impact, 13*(1), 14–15.

Beyond Compliance Coordinating Committee. (n.d.). Retrieved November 21, 2006, from http://bccc.syr.edu/

Blackorby, J., & Wagner, M. (1996). Longitudinal postschool outcomes of youth with disabilities: Findings from the National Longitudinal Transition Study. *Exceptional Children, 62,* 399–413.

Bradley, V., Agosta, J., Smith, G., Taub, S., Ashbaugh, J., Silver, J., & Heaviland, M. (2001). *The Robert Wood Johnson Foundation Self-Determination Initiative: Final impact assessment report.* Cambridge, MA: The Human Services Research Institute.

Developmental Disabilities Bulletin. (1994). Inclusive education services: 7 years of practice. *J.P. Das Developmental Disabilities Centre, 22*(2). Retrieved January 9, 2007, from http://www.ualberta.ca/~jpdasddc/bulletin/22-2-1994.html

Developmental Disabilities Bulletin. (1997). An inclusive university program for students with moderate to severe developmental disabilities: Student, parent, and faculty perspectives. *J.P. Das Developmental Disabilities Centre, 25*(1). Retrieved January 9, 2007, from http://www.ualberta.ca/~jpdasddc/bulletin/25-1-1997.html

Doyle, M.B. (1997). College life: The new frontier. *Impact, 10*(3), 16–17.

Fisher, E. S. (1995). A temporary place to belong: Inclusion in a public speaking and personal relations course. In S.J. Taylor, R. Bogdan, & Z.M. Lutfiyya (Eds.), *The variety of community experience.* Baltimore: Paul H. Brookes Publishing Co.

Frank, S., & Uditsky, B. (1988). On campus: Integration at a university. *Entourage, 3*(3), 111–117.

Fox, K. (2003, February). Two incredible women overcome adversity and attain their goals. *Catholic Sun, 14,* 1–4.

Getzel, E.E., Flippo, K.F., Wittig, K.M., & Russell, D.L. (1997). Beyond high school: Postsecondary education as a transition outcome. In M. Sustrova & S. Pueschel (Eds.), *Adolescents with Down syndrome.* Baltimore: Paul H. Brookes Publishing Co.

Getzel, E.E., & Wehman, P. (2005). *Going to college: Expanding opportunities for people with disabilities.* Baltimore: Paul H. Brookes Publishing Co.

Gilmore, D.S., Schuster, J.L., Timmons, J.C., & Butterworth, J. (2000). Ten years of progress: An analysis of trends for people with mental retardation, cerebral palsy, and epilepsy receiving services from state vocational rehabilitation agencies. *Rehabilitation Counseling Bulletin, 44*(1), 30–39.

Gilmore, D.S., Schuster, J., Zafft, C., & Hart, D. (2001). Postsecondary education services and employment outcomes within the vocational rehabilitation system. *Disability Studies Quarterly, 21*(1), 64–76.

Golden, T., & Jones, M. (2002). Supplemental Security Income and postsecondary education support for students with disabilities. *Impact, 15*(1), 4–5.

Grigal, M., Neubert, D.A., & Moon, M.S. (2001). Public school programs for students with significant disabilities in postsecondary settings. *Education and Training in Mental Retardation and Developmental Disabilities, 36,* 244–254.

Hall, M., Kleinert, H.L., & Kearns, J.F. (2000). Going to college! Postsecondary programs for students with moderate and severe disabilities. *Teaching Exceptional Children, 32*(3), 58–65.

Hamill, L.B. (2003). Going to college: The experience of a young woman with Down syndrome. *Mental Retardation, 41*(5), 340–353.

Hart, D. Zimbrich, K., & Ghiloni, C. (2001). Interagency partnerships and funding individual supports for youth with significant disabilities as they move into postsecondary education and employment options. *Journal of Vocational Rehabilitation, 61*(4), 145–154.

Individuals with Disabilities Education Act of 1990, PL 101-476, 20 U.S.C. §§ 1400 *et seq.*

Individuals with Disabilities Education Improvement Act of 2004, PL 108-446, 20 U.S.C. §§ 1400 *et seq.*

Izzo, M., Hertzfeld, J., Simmons-Reed, E., & Aaron, J. (2001). Promising practices: Improving the quality of higher education for students with disabilities. *Disability Studies Quarterly, 21*(1). Retrieved January 9, 2007, from http://www.cds.hawaii.edu/dsq/winter2001.html

Johnson, D.R., Sharpe, M.N., & Stodden, R.A. (2000). The transition to postsecondary education for students with disabilities. *Impact, 13*(1), 2–3, 26–27.

Johnson, J.L. (n.d.). *Examination of the status of the inclusion of students with developmental disabilities, including significant cognitive disabilities, in postsecondary education* (Findings implications brief). National Center for the Study of Postsecondary Educational Supports, University of Hawaii at Manoa.

Jones, M. (2002). *Providing a quality accommodated experience in preparation for and during postsecondary school* (Information Brief, 1). Minneapolis, MN: National Center on Secondary Education and Transition, Institute on Community Integration, University of Minnesota.

L'Institut Roeher Institute. (1996). *Building bridges: Inclusion in postsecondary education for people with intellectual disabilities.* Toronto: Author.

Luecking, R., & Murphy, S. (2000). Postsecondary options for young adults with intensive support needs. *Impact, 13*(1), 10–11.

National Council on Disability. (2003). *People with disabilities and postsecondary education: Position paper.* Washington, DC: Author.

Neubert, D., Moon, M.S., Grigal, M., & Redd, V. (2001). Postsecondary educational practices for individuals with mental retardation and other significant disabilities: A review of the literature. *Journal of Vocational Rehabilitation, 16*(3,4), 155–168.

Pierangelo, R., & Crane, R. (1997). *Complete guide to special education transition services.* West Nyack, NY: The Center for Applied Research in Education.

Preece, J. (1995). Disability and adult education: The consumer view. *Disability & Society, 10*(1), 87–102.

Rehabilitation Act of 1973, PL 93-112, 29 U.S.C. §§ 31 *et seq.*

Scott, S., McGuire, J., & Shaw, S. (2003). Universal design for instruction: A new paradigm for adult instruction in postsecondary education. *Remedial & Special Education, 24*(6), 369–379.

Seybert, J. (2002, October). Inclusion–Finally! [Keynote speech]. Baltimore: Maryland Coalition for Inclusive Education.

Smith, R. (1997). Varied meanings and practice: Teachers' perspectives regarding high school inclusion. *Journal of The Association for Persons with Severe Handicaps, 22*(4), 235–244.

Stodden, R.A. (2005). The status of persons with disabilities in postsecondary education. *TASH Connections, 2,* 4–5.

U.S. Department of Education National Center for Education Statistics. (1999). *Students with disabilities in postsecondary education: A profile of preparation and outcomes.* Retrieved November 21, 2006, from http://nces.ed.gov/programs/coe/2000/section5/indicator54.asp

Walker, P., Harris, P., Hall, M., Smith, V., & Shoultz, B. (2000). *Self-Determination in Vermont: Contributions of the Vermont Self-Determination Project.* Syracuse, NY: Center on Human Policy.

Weir, C. (2001). Individual supports for college success. *OCO Fact Sheet 7.* Retrieved April 20, 2006, from http://www.education.umd.edu/oco

Yuen, J., & Shaughnessy, B. (n.d.). *Cultural empowerment of students with disabilities in postsecondary education.* Manoa, HI: University of Hawaii National Center for the Study of Postsecondary Educational Supports.

CHAPTER FIVE

Promoting Meaningful Leisure and Social Connections

More than Just Work

PAMELA M. WALKER

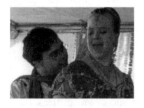

Increasingly, there are opportunities for people with severe developmental disabilities to engage in a variety of meaningful daytime pursuits. This sometimes includes leisure and recreational pursuits, or social connections with friends and neighborhood or community organizations. Social and leisure activities contribute significantly to overall quality and meaningfulness of life (Moon, 1994; Schleien, Ray, & Green, 1997). In addition, social and leisure interests provide opportunities for people to meet others who share interests and possibly form friendships.

This chapter begins with a description of some key components to promoting meaningful leisure and social connections within the overall context of meaningful daytimes. Next, the chapter outlines more specific support strategies in the pursuit of social connections and relationships.

PAID WORK AS A PRIORITY

Like the majority of people without disabilities, most people with severe developmental disabilities desire paid work, so this must be a priority (O'Brien & O'Brien, 2002). When this does not seem to be available, a second priority for many is for education or training that will lead to paid work. At the same time, many people, particularly those with the most severe disabilities, do not have integrated paid work; and many who do have paid work have only a very limited number of hours of paid work per week (Boeltzig, Gilmore, &

Acknowledgment is given to Ann Marie Campbell, Betsy Edinger, Brian Keith, Barbara Prince, Patti Scott, Karlene Shea, Mark Vincent, and Al Zappala for their assistance in the preparation of this chapter.

Butterworth, 2006). Also, when they do have work, they have little choice about this work, resulting in work that may not be meaningful. Thus, for all of these reasons, it is important for many people to have various community connections and engagements, either in addition to or instead of work that can contribute to a meaningful day.

"More than Just a Job"—Meaningful Engagements and Community Connections

Job Path is an agency in New York City that provides inclusive community supports to people with disabilities, including those with severe impairments (Hulgin & Searl, 1996). In the course of the agency's work, agency administrators and staff observed that supported employment services were not meeting the needs of adults with severe disabilities. Job Path was committed to finding ways to support those individuals with the most severe disabilities. They held a retreat and determined that, in order to best meet the needs of people with the most severe disabilities, they needed to shift the focus of their supports beyond just assisting people to find and maintain employment. According to Hulgin and Searl, "People needed opportunities to develop other interests, build social relationships, and in some cases improve their living situations" (1996, p. 6). In turn, these efforts helped create opportunities for employment. For example, some individuals were reluctant to leave the day treatment center for various job opportunities due to lack of social relationships outside the facility. However, over time, as Job Path staff assisted people to develop connections and relationships within their neighborhoods and communities, they became increasingly interested in community employment, and found some job opportunities through these community connections as well.

KEY COMPONENTS IN PROMOTING COMMUNITY CONNECTIONS

Some of the key components in promoting meaningful leisure and community connections include the pursuit of individual interests, access to community places that offer meaningful social contexts, and the opportunity for community connections and social relationships. Underpinning all of these is the element of choice and control with regard to interests, places, and relationships. In this section, each of these areas is discussed.

Pursuit of Individual Interests

John O'Brien and Connie Lyle O'Brien (1987) speak to the importance of interests in adding meaning to one's life as well as in promoting social connection:

> Interests link the personal and the social. They express individual gifts, concerns, and fascinations and call for activities, information, and tools. Shared interest founds association. People point to interests when they describe what gives their lives meaning. (p. 35)

Traditionally, the service system has placed a low priority on leisure and social relationships, and has severely limited the opportunities for people with disabilities to exercise control and choice with regard to pursuit of interests, leisure activities, and social relationships. People with disabilities are increasingly making it clear that they want to have choice and control in their lives. Through individual initiative, with the support of creative agencies, or through alternative support initiatives (e.g., state efforts to promote self-determination through individual budgets, consumer directed supports, support brokers, and the like), people with disabilities are increasingly gaining such opportunities for choice and control regarding meaningful daytimes (Beck, Jupp, & Scott, 2001; Hall & Walker, 1998; Simon, 2002).

Agencies that focus on supported employment/day services as well as those that focus on community living have begun to pay attention to other aspects of people's daytime. Often, over time, they have come to see their agency's mission as being broader than supported employment or residential supports. They have engaged in efforts not only to find work or housing, but to assist people to have broader community engagements and connections based on interest. This includes participation in recreational and leisure activities, neighborhood and community associations, volunteer work, and social relationships (Hall & Walker, 1998; Hulgin & Searl, 1996; Walker, 2000; Walker & Cory, 2002). The following case study describes some benefits of community leisure opportunities.

Craig is a young man with disabilities who receives support from KFI, Inc., a non-profit agency that provides individualized community-based supports in Millinocket, Maine. He lives with his mother. Two brothers have moved out, but live nearby. A community advocate provided support to Craig for 4 hours a day, 5 days a week. One of the primary roles of the community advocate was to help Craig look for a job. Craig was interested in finding a job that involves woodworking. In addition to looking for work, Craig's community advocate has supported him to pursue some leisure interests. For one, he was interested in joining the local gym. Here, Craig began lifting weights, swimming, and taking karate lessons. Over time, he has advanced to the point of serving as a personal trainer for others at the gym, and is working on his brown belt in karate. Craig was also interested in taking guitar lessons. These lessons have led to a close friendship with his guitar teacher. Overall, Craig's involvement in the gym and with his guitar teacher gave him confidence to try other things. One of these was attaining a leadership position in a local self-advocacy group.

Another example illustrates how involvement with a state self-determination project helped one individual make substantial changes in her life based on her interests.

Helen, a middle-age woman with a developmental disability label, was frustrated about lack of a job or other meaningful daytime involvements, and felt that what activities she did have were agency-directed rather than directed by Helen herself. Overall, she felt a lack of control in her life. Helen enlisted the assistance of the State Self-Determination Project, a 3-year initiative to promote increased consumer control and choice, funded by the Robert Wood Johnson Foundation (Aichroth et al., 2002). Helen was interested in gaining more control of her money and exploring different ways of spending it, with the advice and assistance of a team from the self-determination project. Helen's first steps were to request that instead of an exercise program that occupied part of her week, she wanted to use her money to purchase a membership at a health center. In addition, she expressed interest in finding ways to develop her reading and computer skills. These first steps led to many additional choices and opportunities for Helen. Helen chose to maintain agency involvement in provision of her supports, but she made various decisions determining which agency provided support and which individuals provided support. Over time, Helen increased her connections to the self-determination project, and when offered a part-time job with them, she accepted. In addition, Helen increased her involvement with self-advocacy and became involved at the state and national level. At the state level, Helen got involved in the Invisible Victims of Crime Project, which provides education, information, and assistance regarding crime and people with disabilities. She has also been engaged in self-advocacy at the national level. Overall, Helen's life is now filled with involvement in many sorts of activities that are meaningful and important to her.

Importance of Place

An important aspect of a meaningful daytime relates to the place or places where people spend time. People's experience and relationships in certain places vary tremendously; depending on the social context of the places they spend time (Fischer, 1982). In the past, people with developmental disabilities have been denied opportunities for choice about the places they spend time, and often, without their choice or consent, were sent to segregated places designated for individuals with disabilities. They lacked opportunities to establish roots and a sense of belonging within place, as well as opportunity to spend time in shared social spaces with people of their own choosing (O'Brien & O'Brien, 1987; O'Brien & O'Brien, 1992; Walker, 1999).

With increasing deinstitutionalization and development of community-based services, people spend more time within community places (e.g., restaurants, malls, movie theaters, churches, parks, neighborhood centers). However, when supported by the service system to spend time in community places, the places they go tend to be those characterized by a business-transaction oriented context (e.g., malls, theaters), rather than a social orientation (e.g., neighborhood, community organizations), and they are often accompanied there by groups of others with disabilities (Metzel & Walker, 2001; Walker, 1999). Thus, due to the nature of places that people often go, as well as the context in which they go there, they may have only very limited opportunities for social interaction with other community members. However, as people with disabilities gain increasing access to the community, there are times when they become connected to and part of neighborhood and community places that offer social connection and relationship with other community members. This can occur with support from creative agencies, support from family members or friends, support from other community members, or at the person's own initiative (Bartholomew-Lorimer, 1993; Bogdan, 1995; Lutfiyya, 1995; Reidy, 1993). Important attributes of social contexts in which people feel welcome include those places they go of their own choosing where they feel known and accepted, where they feel as if they are full contributing members, and where they receive any support they might need to ensure full participation (Gretz, 1992; Lutfiyya, 1995; O'Brien & O'Brien, 1996; Reidy, 1993; Walker, 1999).

Janice is a woman with a developmental disability who has been a member of the Syracuse Community Choir for about 5 years. The choir is an organization with a mission to be inclusive and diverse. Janice heard about the choir through friends in her self-advocacy group. The choir provides a variety of forms of assistance to Janice to facilitate and enhance her participation. Choir members offer Janice rides to and from rehearsals when needed. Also, it is easier for Janice to read large-print music, and the choir provides this for her. At first, Janice was hesitant about joining a community organization such as the choir, saying, "I didn't know people and I was afraid people would laugh at me." Over time, as she has gotten to know other choir members, she has become very comfortable there. Eventually, she joined the board of directors for the choir. Because it is hard for her to read the typed meeting minutes, the board records the minutes on tape for her. Overall, Janice has found the Syracuse Community Choir is an accepting place for her where she can meet new friends and be a contributing member. Janice now says, "Choir is great. I've met lots of new people and made good friends. Being on the board, I feel like I'm helping the choir out" (Walker, 2001).

Opportunities for Social Relationships and Community Connections

A third aspect critical to meaningful daytimes is social relationships and community connections. All people, including those with disabilities, need enduring, committed, freely chosen relationships (Lutfiyya, 1991; Pitonyak, 2002). Many people with disabilities, particularly those who have spent long years enmeshed in the service system, are cut off from such relationships (Pitonyak, 2002, p. 3). In an effort to remedy this lack of relationship, the Friendship Project was initiated in 1995 through the Philadelphia Office of Mental Health and Mental Retardation based on the recognition that some individuals with developmental disabilities who lived in the community still experienced significant social isolation (Mount, 1995; O'Brien, 1996). As one of the founders described,

> We designed the Friendship Project because we found that even when person-centered plans had been done, people had better lives and were realizing their dreams, but the missing piece was community. A lot of times people just didn't focus on that, it fell by the wayside. So people were still surrounded by paid staff and other people with disabilities. (A.M. Campbell, personal communication, 2003)

Central to this effort was the recognition that people needed various types of relationships and social connections, including an inner circle of close relationships, as well as an outer circle of additional friendships and community connections (Mount, 1995; O'Brien & O' Brien, 1996). One person assisted by the Friendship Project was Rob, who was not content with his life.

Rob is 40 years old and is labeled with a developmental disability. His parents attributed his lack of contentment to a number of things, including his dissatisfaction with life in a group home, his dissatisfaction spending days at a sheltered workshop, and his general dissatisfaction due to lack of friends and meaningful activities. His parents enlisted the assistance of the Friendship Project. Together, they formed a circle of support for Rob. A circle of support is a framework that has been used to assist individuals with developmental disabilities to identify dreams and desires and to achieve these (O'Brien & O'Brien, 1996). It involves convening a core group of committed people to assist a given individual, with emphasis on involvement of those who are not just paid staff (Mount, Beeman, & Ducharme, 1988; Pearpoint, 1990).

Over the years, the circle of support has assisted Rob in changing many aspects of his life for the better. He now lives in his own apartment with 24-hour support. A job coach helped him try out a number of different kinds of jobs, in search of one that would be a good match for Rob. A couple of days a week, he does office work for the agency that supports him; two other days a week, he has a job at a store. This seems to be a good match for Rob, who had grown up spending time around the store that his parents' owned. In his free time, Rob spends a lot of time with family members. However, his circle of support has also helped connect him to other community members based on his interests. He enjoys riding bikes with a friend and has become a member of a neighborhood association, as well as joining the local YMCA. Rob is also taking reading lessons. While the circle of support has often worked collaboratively with the agency that supports Rob, the circle of support has served as a force to push where the agency was not taking action or was contemplating action that was possibly detrimental to Rob's well-being. For instance, Rob has a strong preference for living on his own. At times agency staff has discussed the possibility of placing a roommate in Rob's apartment; at these times, his circle members have adamantly advocated with agency staff and administrators about the importance of Rob living in his own place.

Within the broad framework discussed above of interests, community places, and social relationships, there are many varied strategies being utilized to help promote meaningful leisure and social opportunities for individuals with disabilities. The following section describes some of these strategies.

STRATEGIES WITHIN AND BEYOND THE SERVICE SYSTEM FOR PROMOTING LEISURE AND SOCIAL CONNECTIONS

This section of the chapter reviews numerous approaches and strategies in promoting leisure and social connections. These include 1) creative approaches that are being used within human service agencies, 2) self-determination initiatives, 3) in-depth individualized planning and circles of support, 4) other service system and community initiatives, and 5) individual initiatives.

Creative Agency Approaches

Agencies that provide day services as well as those that provide residential services can use a variety of strategies to promote leisure opportunities and community connections as a broader part of efforts to ensure meaningful daytimes for adults with disabilities. Such strategies include 1) supporting people's lives as a whole, 2) reliance on the community versus a facility, 3) alternative uses of day services funding, and 4) placing renewed emphasis on collaboration with families. Each strategy is described in this chapter. This is by no means an exhaustive set of strategies, but serves to illustrate some of the options and approaches that are available to support agencies.

Supporting People's Lives as a Whole   Traditionally, services for people with disabilities have been segmented, and individuals often receive residential supports from one agency, employment or day services from another, and so forth. In order to support people to have meaningful daytimes, and more broadly, meaningful lives, some agencies have found it more effective to move in the direction of seeing people's lives as a whole; and coordinating and combining funding and supports for day, residential, and other services (Hall & Walker, 1998; Walker, 1999).

For example, at Common Ground, an agency in Littleton, New Hampshire, agency staff were concerned about the segmentation of support services. They have taken a variety of steps to address this. They revised the agency's mission statement to incorporate the importance of addressing people's lives as a whole, and they established greater collaboration between staff involved in case management, employment/day supports, and supported living, These changes, among others, have led to new ways of assisting people such as Emily.

Emily, an outgoing woman, is 35 years old and has been labeled as having mental retardation. On the surface, it appeared as though her life was fine, as she was living in a "developmental home" (i.e., family care) with a family who were committed to her and who assisted her to participate in a variety of community places and activities. In the past, Emily lived with her mother for most of her life, until her mother became too elderly to provide the assistance that Emily needed. Since that time, Emily lived with various family care providers, the most recent being the current living situation, in a very rural setting. Thus, Emily was dependent on the family for transportation to participate in community events and activities. Emily expressed her desire to move; in particular, she wanted her own apartment close to the center of a small town that she was familiar with. Emily's mother, and Emily's siblings, after her mother's death, all favored life with a family care provider for Emily. Agency staff helped Emily convince her siblings about the importance of Emily's choice in this matter and provided information about the safeguards that would be in place (e.g., security systems within the apartment building, agency emergency contact measures). Emily now has her own apartment within a small complex. Day services staff and residential services staff from the agency have worked together with Emily to develop meaningful work and other engagements in her life. Two days a week, she assists with office work at her apartment complex. For a long time, Emily wanted to be a secretary, so the opportunity for this type of work is important to her. Also, 2 days a week, she volunteers at a nearby nursing home. In her spare time, she enjoys taking part in some of the organized activities within the apartment complex, such as bingo, potlucks, and trips. In addition, she walks to the local library, church, stores, and community pancake dinners. There is a community bus that she uses for trips to her foot doctor. A support staff person spends about 25 hours a week with Emily. In addition to banking and other business, Emily and the support staff person swim together three times a week. In addition to this staff person, two other staff from the agency live nearby and check in on her. Also, there is emergency assistance available through her apartment complex if the need arises. Some old family friends welcome her for holidays and other celebrations. Emily also travels to visit her siblings in other parts of the country. Overall, with this change in her life, Emily is now able to exercise significant control in determining her involvement in various community places, events, and social networks within her community.

Reliance on the Community versus on a Facility

Just as place is significant for individuals, so, too, are the spaces and/or places that community agencies occupy. The sorts of spaces and places that are occupied by community agencies play a critical role in defining community participation for the people they support. A small but increasing number of agencies are closing sheltered workshops and day habilitation centers and choosing to provide supports to everyone within the community versus reliance on a facility (Hall & Walker, 1998; Murphy & Rogan, 1995; Walker, 1999). This requires new staff roles focused on assisting people to find community employment and other meaningful daytime engagements. And, it entails forging new relationships with the community.

Common Ground closed its sheltered workshops in 1994. Since that time, as part of the effort to help people find community employment, it has been part of the job of all staff to form community connections and to assist the people they support to develop community connections. While these community connections have been important in and of themselves, they have also been important to helping people find and keep jobs. For instance, in assisting a young man, Tim, to find a job, it was Tim's relationship with a woman who works at one of the local banks, originally fostered through agency staff, that was instrumental in helping him find the type of job he desired, that is, working at a McDonald's that is close to his apartment. One of the agency staff members reflected,

> The day I knew we had a success story in the making was when I heard how he is telling everyone he got the job on his own, and it's that sense of ownership that's sustaining him right now when things go wrong at work.

Use of Daytime Funding in Alternative Ways   Neighbours, Inc., is a nonprofit corporation based in Franklin Park, New Jersey. As stated on their web site, this organization "has been formed for the sole purpose of enabling people who have disabilities to have a full and exciting life within their local communities" (Neighbours, Inc., n.d.). Neighbours, Inc., provides assistance to people across a wide variety of areas including housing and support services; employment and other meaningful daytime pursuits; and the development of relationships and circles of support (Walker & Cory, 2002). Regarding day services, the agency has helped numerous individuals move from traditional day services (e.g., sheltered employment, day habilitation) to community jobs and other meaningful daytime pursuits. Some people they support are clear about what they would like to do—for instance, one young man moved from a nursing home into his own apartment. He is an artist, creating hand-painted and computer-designed cards that he sells at craft fairs and on the Internet. His advisor from Neighbours, Inc., helps him with development and management of his business and with connections to others in the arts community.

Another woman who was assisted by Neighbours, Inc., is Lila. Lila made it clear
to others that she no longer wanted to go to a senior day program. Lila was 78 years
old, and had lived in an institution for 50 years. Neighbours, Inc., assisted her to
move to a house in the same town as her brother. The agency did not have funding
for day services for Lila, but was committed to using other financial resources from
within the agency in order to support her choice to not attend the senior day pro-
gram. As the agency director put it, "When you're 80 years old, no one should
make you go somewhere you don't want to because they don't have money for an
alternative" (Walker & Cory, 2002, p. 12). So, instead, the agency assisted Lila to
spend the days of her last year of life pursuing hobbies and interests that were special
to her—that is, caring for her numerous pets (a cat, a dog, a rabbit, some birds, and a
turtle), and going to pet shows, flower shows, arts and crafts fairs, and other commu-
nity events.

Other people are not as clear about what type of job they would like and what other interests they might like to pursue due to lack of previous knowledge about or exposure to community options. Therefore, support may involve significant time for exploration.

A woman named Martha lived in an institution from the time she was
6 years old until she was 32. In the institution, she often expressed her anger and
frustration in ways that were harmful to herself and others. Because of this, when the
institution closed, Martha was considered dangerous and it was likely that she would
be sent to a locked group home. However, her state-appointed guardian strongly felt
that congregate residential or day services would be very detrimental to Martha. As
an alternative, her guardian helped her obtain support from Neighbours, Inc., to live
in her own apartment with 24-hour support. The funding provided for Martha was
not quite sufficient to meet her needs, so Neighbours, Inc., supplemented her budget

in order to provide supports rather than forcing her to go to a workshop or day habili-tation center. Since she has been living in her own place, Martha has far fewer occa-sions of intense anger. She is much more comfortable around people and her network of friends is expanding. Martha enjoys baking, so Trish, an agency staff person, has assisted Martha to find or create work that involves baking.

Collaboration with Families   In recent years, there have been efforts both within the system and beyond the system to promote greater oppor-tunities for real choice for individuals with developmental disabilities. When these individuals live with family members or have significant family involvement, there may be both commonalities and differences between the person's interests and those of the family. When support agencies assist individuals with disabilities, particularly with regard to differing interests, a key factor is the agency's relationship with families.

Joe, who is in his late 30s, lives with his aging parents, who are highly protective of him. He has never worked and has been involved in very little outside the home, as his parents fear he will be taken advantage of. He tried a day habilitation program for about a year and a half. In this program, Joe was grouped with other individuals with disabilities for various activities and community outings. However, this did not work for Joe, who does not want to spend his days with groups of others based on disabil-ity. It was evident to Joe's service coordinator at a human services agency in Syracuse, New York, that Joe would benefit from involvement in some sort of activity, rather than just sitting home day after day. During previous conversations with the service coordinator, Joe expressed an interest in karate, so the coordinator approached his parents about this possibility. Though hesitant, their willingness to let Joe try karate was based on their long-term, trusting relationship. The coordinator accompa-nied him to sign up; then, his parents drove him for the first couple of months. Since that time, his parents have been unable to drive him, due to health problems, so the service coordinator arranged transportation using state family support funds. Joe has since worked up to his brown belt in karate and also spends some of his time at home now practicing karate. Based on this positive experience, Joe's parents have been receptive to the initiation of other community activities. For example, Joe had a long-standing interest in reading, and he now meets with a tutor from Literacy Volunteers twice a week at the public library. Again, this is another activity in which he can engage at home.

Self-Determination

When individuals receive services provided through an agency, there are often limitations to the degree of control and choice regarding daytime options. Though not without any limitations, self-determination initiatives within vari-ous states have expanded the available options. Individuals who in the past were offered only sheltered employment, day habilitation, menial jobs, or nothing, have been able to design creative employment options, including self-employment, as well as pursue other community interests and connections. The case studies in this section illustrate the positive effects of self-determination.

Through Philadelphia's self-determination project, which incorporated the use of support brokers, Sam was liberated from a life that was controlled by the service system. Previously, Sam lived in a large institution, then a 3-person group home, which he considered to be in many ways similar to an institution in terms of control of his life. He now lives in his own apartment, and is looking for work. He is also interested in going back to school and then to college. He hires his own personal care assistants and now he has the freedom to determine his own daily schedule rather than have an agency dictate many aspects of this. One of his priorities is involvement with ADAPT; others include visits with his mom, his girlfriend, traveling, and shopping.

Mark previously lived in an institution, then in a group home. He experienced severe abuse in the institution; he had significant difficulties in the group home as well, and engaged in self-destructive behaviors (A.M. Campbell, 2003, personal communication; Pitonyak, 2002). A group of people who had known Mark over time met with him to express their concerns over his well-being. Mark said to them, "I want my life back" (A.M. Campbell, 2003, personal communication). This group of people committed themselves to standing by Mark and supporting him to pursue this objective. They helped Mark become part of Philadelphia's self-determination initiative. This enabled him to gain significant control of his life, so he could select his support staff and determine the ways in which he would spend his time. Self-determination has had its challenges for Mark; for instance, he has had difficulties finding and keeping good staff. Mark's support broker and circle of support are providing support in managing his staff. Overall, the self-determination initiative has provided three critical things in Mark's life. First, he is now in control. Second, he has a sense of trust and belonging with a committed circle of people who have supported his self-determination. Third, on the basis of his sense of control, trust, and belonging, Mark is now able to explore important interests in his life; two of the major ones include gardening and spending time at a radio station.

Individualized Planning and Circles of Support

Individualized planning (e.g., person-centered planning, Making Action Plans [MAPs], essential lifestyle planning) and circles of support have been very useful in helping many individuals to build and sustain meaningful lives (O'Brien & O'Brien, 1996; 2002). Such planning and support is characterized by a group of people who are committed to assisting a particular individual to create desired change in his or her life. Increasingly, service agencies are attempting to incorporate various aspects of individualized planning. However, there are often limitations to such agency-based planning, as they often are dominated by service system staff and do not incorporate enough emphasis on enduring community connections and participation and, also, it can be very difficult for these staff members to advocate for substantive change in the person's services (Lutfiyya, 1993). In contrast, in Philadelphia, in 1989, the Personal Futures Planning Project was initiated in order to assist some individuals who were most vulnerable to making changes in their lives, including increased social networks and community participation, with the involvement of individuals who were not paid agency support staff in planning; these individuals were committed to forming long-term relationships, helping them establish other community connections, and advocating on the person's behalf (Alimena-Caruso & Lee, 2000; Mount, 1995; O'Brien, 1996).

Rose, a resilient woman in her late 60s, is labeled with a significant developmental disability. A circle of support was formed for Rose because her life was in chaos (Alimena-Caruso & Lee, 2000). She had a reputation for being challenging to support, and engaged in a significant amount of behavior that was harmful to herself. Consequently, she often spent a large part of her day in a "time-out room" at her group home. Her support agency was so challenged by her behavior that they were considering sending her back to an institution. Members of the Personal Futures Planning Project who knew Rose feared for her life, particularly if she was reinstitutionalized. So, as part of this project, they initiated a circle of support around her. They began by listening. However, Rose is not a person who is verbally expressive and could not just tell her life story. Members of the Personal Futures Planning Project attempted to listen to who she was by being with her and by piecing together what others wrote about her in the past. What this process revealed was, among other things, how socially isolated and disconnected she was. She had no family. She had no one in her life except those who were paid to be there, and they never stayed connected to her over the long term. Also, there was no one she could trust in her life.

Members of the circle of support have played multiple roles in Rose's life. Perhaps most importantly, they developed trusting, committed, long-term relationships with her. This occurred over time, particularly as they regularly spent time with her, made various commitments to her, and stood by those commitments. Circle members have also assisted Rose to develop some meaningful daytime routines based on her interest and choice. Finally, circle members have assisted agency staff to create supports for Rose that promote her choice and control and that promote meaningful community experiences and connections.

Special Initiatives

Across the country, there have been some notable special initiatives designed to promote meaningful neighborhood and community participation and social connections. Though these are not targeted toward people's daytimes, in particular, they encompass activities and relationships that include daytime hours and engagements. Such initiatives have been established both by disability organizations as well as community organizations.

In both Pennsylvania and Massachusetts, the state developmental disabil-ities planning councils have funded projects aimed at assisting individuals with disabilities to become members of community associations (Gretz, 1992; Reidy, 1993).

A disabled man named George has been a member of the Knights of Columbus, in Chicopee, Massachusetts, since 1988 (K. Shea, personal communication, 2006). Aside from work at an office 2 days a week, George spends much of his time at the Knights of Columbus hall. "Before the Knights, most of his free time was either spent watch-ing television or riding his three-wheel bicycle up and down the street near his house" (Reidy, 1993, p. 353). Now, George's life is filled with activities and friend-ships made through the Knights of Columbus. He contributes greatly to the organiza-tion, helping out at weekly bingo, monthly meetings, dinners, and other events. George's relationships with the Knights extend beyond organizational events, and friends from the organization invite him to their homes, assist him with odd jobs at his home, and help him visit and tend his parents' graves, among other things. Overall, as a result of his involvement with the Knights, George now is very engaged in his community and has an extensive network of friends and acquaintances.

In the state of Washington, "Involving All Neighbors" was initiated by a community organization, the Seattle Department of Neighborhoods; it is a col-laborative project with the Washington State Division of Developmental Disabilities (Carlson, 2000). Through this project, there were many lessons learned about involving people in neighborhood organizations. For human service agencies, some of the lessons were about the importance of finding a match for the person's interests; the importance of finding valued roles for peo-ple; that support could be generated for people, but it most often came through relationships; and that building relationships takes time.

Individual Initiatives

Recognition must be given to the power of people with disabilities to create meaningful daytimes for themselves, without the assistance of agencies, or specially designed initiatives or projects. Often, these are people who are dis-satisfied with the options they have been offered by the system and want to minimize system involvement in their lives. For instance, in *Riding the Bus with My Sister,* Rachael Simon (2002) writes poignantly about her sister's rejection of system alternatives and her creation of her own meaningful daytime routines and relationships. Simon points to the importance of viewing what constitutes a meaningful daytime on an individual-by-individual basis. In addition, she discusses dilemmas balancing concerns about her sister's safety and well-being with her sister's right to choice and self-determination.

Another example is provided by a man named Zach, who formerly lived in an insti-tution and then a group home. He now has a room in a small boarding house. Through his own initiative, he has created a variety of meaningful daytime engage-

ments for himself. Zach spends a lot of time in his neighborhood walking around chatting with people, collecting bottles, and doing odd jobs such as stump removal and other yard work. By word of mouth, demand for Zach's work has grown. As he walks the neighborhood in between jobs, or before and after, he chats with people on the street and in the local coffee shops. Through his contacts with people at the university, dropping by to visit, word spread about his expertise in math. In addition to his yard work, he now regularly presents to math classes at Syracuse University, and occasionally presents at conferences and other forums.

CONCLUSION

Leisure activities as well as community connections and social relationships can be a critical part of a meaningful daytime. This is particularly true for those individuals who, for whatever reason, do not have paid employment or do not have many regular hours of paid employment. Within the service system, it can be the role of either or both a residential support services staff or a day support services staff to assist individuals to seek meaningful daytime opportunities and engagements. In the past, service systems have posed significant barriers to community connections. Increasingly, there are examples of agencies that provide creative support for meaningful daytimes. There are, however, limitations to the extent that the service system can foster meaningful connections and relationships in people's lives. Individualized planning and support processes, self-determination initiatives, and other special efforts of human service organizations and community members can help enhance connections and opportunities, offering choice and control, flexibility, and support from those who are not paid staff. At the same time, important recognition needs to be given to people's own initiative in creating meaningful daytimes for themselves.

Meaningful daytime engagements that relate to leisure and social relationships have many benefits. They can lead to opportunities to obtain paid employment, as well as support to maintain employment. In addition, meaningful daytime pursuits can make a substantial contribution to improving the quality of people's lives and their sense of community membership and participation.

REFERENCES

Aichroth, S., Carpenter, J., Daniels, K., Grassette, P., Kelly, D., Murray, A., et al. (2002). Creating a new system of supports: The Vermont Self-Determination Project. *Rural Special Education Quarterly, 21*(2), 16–28.

Alimena-Caruso, M., & Lee, K. (2000). *Stories of the glories of person-centered planning and circles of support.* Harrisburg, PA: Pennsylvania Developmental Disabilities Council.

Amado, A.N. (1993). Steps for supporting community connections. In A.N. Amado (Ed.), *Friendships and community connections between people with and without disabilities* (pp. 299–326). Baltimore: Paul H. Brookes Publishing Co.

Bartholomew-Lorimer, K. (1993). Community building: Valued roles for supporting connections. In A.N. Amado (Ed.), *Friendships and community connections between people with and without developmental disabilities* (pp. 169–180). Baltimore: Paul H. Brookes Publishing Co.

Beck, K., Jupp, K., & Scott, P. (2001). *The support broker's manual*. Franklin Park, NJ: Art of the Possible Publications.

Boeltzig, H., Gilmore, D.S., & Butterworth, J. (2006). The national survey of community rehabilitation providers FY2004–2005 report 1: Employment outcomes of people with developmental disabilities in integrated employment. *Research and Practice, 44*.

Bogdan, R. (1995). Singing for an inclusive society: The Syracuse Community Choir. In S.J. Taylor, R. Bogdan, & Z.M. Lutfiyya (Eds.), *The variety of community experience: Qualitative studies of family and community life*. Baltimore: Paul H. Brookes Publishing Co.

Carlson, C. (2000). *Involving all neighbors: Building inclusive communities in Seattle*. Seattle: City of Seattle Department of Neighborhoods.

Fischer, C.S. (1982). *To dwell among friends: Personal networks in town and city*. Chicago: The University of Chicago Press.

Gretz, S. (1992). Citizen participation: Connecting people to associational life. In D.B. Schwartz (Ed.), *Crossing the river: Creating a conceptual revolution in community & disability*. Cambridge, MA: Brookline Books.

Hall, M., & Walker, P. (1998). *This is still a work in progress*. Syracuse, NY: Center on Human Policy.

Hulgin, K., & Searl, J. (1996). *Job Path: Shifting the focus beyond just work*. Syracuse, NY: Center on Human Policy.

Lutfiyya, Z.M. (1991). A feeling of being connected: Friendships between people with and without learning disabilities. *Disability, Handicap, & Society, 6*(3), 233–245.

Lutfiyya, Z.M. (1993). When "staff" and "clients" become friends. In A.N. Amado (Ed.), *Friendships and community connections between people with and without developmental disabilities* (pp. 97–108). Baltimore: Paul H. Brookes Publishing Co.

Lutfiyya, Z.M. (1995). Baking bread together: A study of membership and inclusion. In S.J. Taylor, R. Bogdan, & Z.M. Lutfiyya (Eds.), *The variety of community experiences: Qualitative studies of family and community life*. Baltimore: Paul H. Brookes Publishing Co.

Metzel, D., & Walker, P. (2001, Fall). The illusion of inclusion: Geographies of the lives of people with developmental disabilities in the United Sates. *Disability Studies Quarterly, 21*(4).

Moon, M.S. (1994). (Ed.) *Making school and community recreation fun for everyone: Places and ways to integrate*. Baltimore: Paul H. Brookes Publishing Co.

Mount, B. (1995). *Building connections to the wheel of relationship and community life*. Philadelphia: Office of Mental Health and Mental Retardation.

Mount, B., Beeman, P., & Ducharme, G. (1988). *What are we learning about circles of support?* Manchester, CT: Communitas, Inc.

Murphy, S.T., & Rogan, P.M. (1995). *Closing the shop*. Baltimore: Paul H. Brookes Publishing Co.

Neighbours, Inc. (n.d.). *What we are about*. Retrieved November 20, 2006, from http://www.neighborsmn.org

O'Brien, J. (1996). *The Friendship Project: Community building in Philadelphia*. Philadelphia: Office of Mental Health and Mental Retardation.

O'Brien, J., & O'Brien, C.L. (1987). *Framework for accomplishment*. Lithonia, GA: Responsive Systems Associates.

O'Brien, J. & O'Brien, C.L. (1992). *Members of other: Building community in company with people with developmental disabilities*. Toronto: Inclusion Press.

O'Brien, J., & O'Brien, C.L. (1996). *Members of each other*. Toronto: Inclusion Press.

O'Brien, J., & O'Brien, C.L. (2002). *Beating the odds: People with severe and profound disabilities as a resource in the development of supported employment*. Lithonia, GA: Responsive Systems Associates.

Pearpoint, J. (1990). *From behind the piano: The building of Judith's Shaw's unique circle of friends*. Toronto: Inclusion Press.

Pitonyak, D. (2002). Opening the door. In J. O'Brien & C.L. O'Brien, *Implementing person-centered planning: Voices of experience*. Toronto: Inclusion Press.

Reidy, D. (1993). Friendship and community associations. In A.N. Amado (Ed.), *Friendships and community connections between people with and without developmental disabilities* (pp. 351–372). Baltimore: Paul H. Brookes Publishing Co.

Schleien, S.J., Ray, M.T., & Green, F.P. (Eds.). (1997). *Community recreation and people with disabilities: Strategies for inclusion.* Baltimore: Paul H. Brookes Publishing Co.

Simon, R. (2002). *Riding the bus with my sister.* New York: Houghton Mifflin.

Walker, P. (1999). From community presence to sense of place: Community experiences of adults with developmental disabilities. *Journal of The Association for Persons with Severe Handicaps, 24*(1), 23–32.

Walker, P. (2000). *Acting on a vision: Agency conversation at KFI, Millinocket, Maine.* Syracuse, NY: Center on Human Policy.

Walker, P. (2001). Singing for social justice. *Impact, 14* (2), 15, 27.

Walker, P., & Cory, R. (2002). *Shifting from empowered agencies to empowered people.* Syracuse, NY: Center on Human Policy.

CHAPTER SIX

Advocacy and Systems Change Work

PAMELA M. WALKER, PERRY WHITTICO, AND BONNIE SHOULTZ

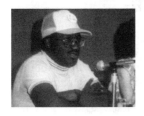

Over the past several years, an increasing amount of people with developmental disabilities have demanded and gained more control and choice in their lives (Bradley et al., 2001; Lakin & Turnbull, 2005). As a result, they are interested in helping other people with disabilities advocate for more control and choice, and in helping to make changes in the service system that promote increased choice and control. Through the self-advocacy movement, as well as other initiatives related to self-determination, growing numbers of people with developmental disabilities are seeking to do advocacy and systems change work on a regular, weekly basis, as a paid job. The expansion of the self-advocacy network itself has created more leadership opportunities, some of which are in paid positions (Self Advocates Becoming Empowered [SABE], 2004). In addition, the expansion of the self-advocacy movement has influenced other organizations (e.g., state mental retardation/developmental disabilities services offices, state developmental disabilities councils, national mental retardation/developmental disabilities advocacy organizations) and initiatives (e.g., the Robert Wood Johnson Foundation's state self-determination projects) to involve people with disabilities in key positions (Powers et al., 2002). This chapter focuses on self-advocates in paid self-advocacy and systems change work. In doing so, it does not focus on the critically important role of the volunteer self-advocacy work that all of those who were interviewed also engaged in. The chapter is based on qualitative interviews with seven self-advocates who have had paid employment related to self-advocacy and systems change.

BACKGROUND TO THE SELF-ADVOCACY MOVEMENT

The first self-advocacy organization in the United States was People First of Oregon, established in 1970. In the early days of the self-advocacy movement, all of the work of establishing and maintaining local and statewide self-advocacy networks was on a volunteer basis. Nebraska formed a statewide organization in the early 1980s (Ward & Shoultz, 2000). As Nancy Ward describes,

> Our local self-advocacy groups grew and we formed People First of Nebraska early in the 1980s. All of us, the members and the advisors, were involved as volunteers. None of us were paid. Then we got some grant money from Nebraska Advocacy Services, enough to hire a staff person. The People First of Nebraska Board of Directors hired me as their Self-Advocacy Organizer, and I worked 20 hours a week with them until January of 1997. I was the only staff person, and our office was my bedroom. (p. 178)

By the late 1970s and early 1980s, many state organizations had been established (Dybwad & Bersani, 1996). Then, at the First North American Self-Advocacy convention in September 1990, plans were put in place that would lead to the development of the national self-advocacy organization, SABE, which was officially established in 1991 (Whittico & Ingram, 1994). Overarching objectives of SABE include 1) promoting legislation at the state and national levels; 2) realizing self-advocacy is hard work and the need to support one another and to celebrate victories; 3) building coalitions; 4) providing public education and awareness; 5) supporting existing state and local organizations, to help start new organizations and to link all self-advocacy organizations; 6) providing resources and training for people with disabilities, advisors, and other people; 7) sharing ideas and information among groups to learn from one another; and 8) identifying funding sources and getting money to fund the national organization (Shoultz & Ward, 1996). Some of SABE's more specific goals include 1) making self-advocacy available in every state including institutions, high schools, rural areas, and people living with families with local support and advisors to help; 2) working with the criminal justice system and people with disabilities about their rights within the criminal justice system; 3) closing institutions for people with developmental disabilities labels nationwide; and 4) building community supports (SABE, 1994). As an organization, SABE members advocate in a multitude of ways, including the production of written, audio, and video materials; sponsorship and participation in conferences, trainings, meetings, and other forums, and so on. SABE advocates on its own, as well as in conjunction with other groups and organizations. For example, SABE joined with ADAPT, a national activist organization (e.g., fighting for accessibility and community-based attendant services; http://www.adapt.org) and the National Council of Independent Living Centers in issuing a "Statement of Solidarity" regarding disability rights and services (Powers et al., 2002).

This expansion, in numbers, organization, and influence, of the self-advocacy network has created opportunities for self-advocates to work on a part- or full-time basis in paid positions. This encompasses work with local, state, and national self-advocacy and cross-disability advocacy organizations; state systems change initiatives; advocacy positions for state or regional developmental disabilities offices and organizations; and university research centers.

The first part of this chapter focuses on the experiences and perspectives of self-advocates who do paid self-advocacy or systems change work. It describes how they became involved in paid work; what types of work they do; and their perspectives regarding some of the positive aspects and challenges to their work. A concluding section discusses some ways that other organizations and entities can engage in genuine collaboration with self-advocates.

SELF-ADVOCACY AND SYSTEMS CHANGE WORK

Growing up as an African American, Perry often experienced a sense of injustice and unequal rights. For example, as he put it, "When I was little and went into a store, and I had my $5 and someone else had his, and I get pushed to the back of the line, cause he's got lighter skin. At some point, you say, wait a minute, this isn't right, but that usually got you into trouble."

Later, as an adult, since moving out of his mother's home, he has relied in part on services from the disability services system due to a learning disability and mental health diagnosis. In this system, too, he has experienced injustices.

> Actually, I think nobody has rights in the service system. The workers are always trying to conform to one model which is given to them by their supervisors. There's always a door, or hallway, or window, or something, that keeps the workers and people apart. And no one ever stops to think that the barrier is always there.

Perry sees some parallels between people who get involved in advocacy related to civil rights issues and people who get involved in self-advocacy related to disability issues. He feels people do not become advocates unless they first recognize the sense of injustice or a lack of rights. Then, he notices two responses. "People get pushed down and do nothing, or people start fighting for their rights." Perry explains that at first he "went into the corner and did nothing." Finally, he says, "What got me started fighting for my rights was the idea that if you didn't fight at all, your rights would go down farther and farther."

Eventually, Perry grew tired of inaction. He got involved in self-advocacy in 1984 after going to a conference sponsored by a local self-advocacy group. At the conference, he met some of the leaders of that group as well as some of the advisors; he volunteered to help during the conference, and after the conference he decided to continue his involvement with Self-Advocates of Central New York.

After being part of this group for a few years, Perry eventually became involved with self-advocacy at the state and national levels. Perry was on the board of SABE from 1992 through 1996. These years were a time during which much of the focus was on creating an organization (e.g., deciding organizational structure, mission) and team-building. It was exciting but challenging work. Perry found the travel for both state and national meetings to be stressful, and he decided to focus his energy back on the local level. Soon after this, he moved into a part-time paid position (approximately 16 hours a month) with the Grassroots Regional Organizing Project (GROP), funded by the Self-Advocacy Association of New York to promote and support the development of local self-advocacy groups. In addition, he had a part-time paid position (approximately 20 hours a month) for OnBoard, a project promoting board and committee membership funded by the state developmental disabilities planning council. At the same time, he continued with volunteer participation in some local and state self-advocacy committees and events.

Pathways to Involvement in Advocacy Work

All of the individuals who were interviewed for this chapter first became involved in organized self-advocacy at the local level and on a volunteer basis. All names are pseudonyms, except the co-author Perry Whittico, as the intent is to provide examples rather than to tell people's stories. There were two major factors that led to their involvement in self-advocacy: 1) They had a sense of injustice regarding the way they and others are treated by society, and 2) their personal networks or the influence of other key people led them to become involved in self-advocacy. After their initial experience and development of leadership skills at the local level, they decided to pursue self-advocacy work further, on a volunteer and paid basis, in regional, state, and national self-advocacy efforts.

Sense of Injustice   Similar to Perry, most if not all of the self-advocates experienced problems within the service system and in society on a broader level. They also witnessed the problems of others. This led to a sense of injustice, which prompted their involvement in self-advocacy. Ann has been involved in self-advocacy for over 20 years. In her past, Ann experienced segregation within special education programs as well as in sheltered workshops. She felt that, based on her disability label, she was denied opportunities to pursue various educational and career paths, as well as being denied opportunities to apply for certain jobs. These experiences contributed to her motivation to get involved in self-advocacy: "I felt I was being discriminated against, and I saw other people who were being discriminated against." Fred, another self-advocate, said he was motivated to get involved in advocacy work because of dissatisfaction with his day services. He was attending a segregated day habilitation facility and felt trapped there. As he describes, "It was hard for anyone to get out of the place, even for part of the day. It was even harder for me and others with wheelchairs."

Personal Network and Influence of Key People   In addition to being motivated by a sense of injustice, people got involved in self-advocacy through personal networks. The influence and invitation of other people helped recruit people initially to do volunteer advocacy work, and also helped encourage them to pursue further self-advocacy work. Hannah, for example, was motivated to get involved in self-advocacy by the example of family members who had been involved in community and political issues, as well as by the invitation and support of other self-advocates. As a teenager, Hannah's parents placed her in a segregated residential school. It was there that she first joined a self-advocacy group. After initial experience at the local level, she was encouraged by other self-advocates and friends to pursue involvement in self-advocacy at the state and national levels. Similar to Hannah, other people we interviewed mentioned getting involved in self-advocacy due to the influence of other self-advocates and at the invitation of self-advocacy advisors. For example, Fred mentioned that "seeing the pride of other self-advocates" convinced him to get involved.

Development of Leadership Skills at Regional, State, and National Levels   All of those who were interviewed started doing self-advocacy work in a volunteer capacity. As a result of their involvement in local self-advocacy, they began to develop leadership skills and experience and were interested in further development of these skills at statewide and national levels, both through volunteer and paid positions. For example, Hannah began her involvement in self-advocacy in a group at the residential school where she lived. Soon, she moved into a leadership position within this group. Next, Hannah became active at the state level, as a member of a consumer advisory board. Later, she began work at the national level, serving on national boards and committees concerned with self-advocacy issues and disability issues more broadly.

Types of Self-Advocacy Work

Though opportunities for paid advocacy and systems change work are not widespread, people with developmental disabilities are increasingly becoming involved in diverse paid work related to self-advocacy and systems change at the local, state, and national levels. This includes work for self-advocacy organizations, state developmental disabilities services offices, grant projects at university research centers, and other types of organizations (Administration for Children and Families, 2004; National Center for the Dissemination of Disability Research [NCDDR], 2003; SABE, 2004). Most of the individuals interviewed for this chapter work for self-advocacy organizations, while some work for other organizations. This section describes some aspects of their work.

Self-Advocacy Organizations   As the self-advocacy movement has expanded, and organizations have grown, particularly at the regional and state level, some have acquired the ability to hire paid workers. This is typically part-time work, funded through a variety of sources, such as state developmental disabilities offices, state developmental disabilities councils, and various grants. For example, while state developmental disabilities councils have a long record of support for self-advocacy, as of 2000, it is law (e.g., the Developmental Disabilities Assistance and Bill of Rights Act of 1975 [PL 94-103]) that all councils provide some direct funding to a state self-advocacy organization led by individuals with developmental disabilities (National Association of Councils on Developmental Disabilities, 2005).

Ann works as a self-advocacy coordinator for a state self-advocacy organization. It is a 40-hour a week position, funded through the local Arc. One of her primary responsibilities is supporting 13 statewide self-advocacy chapters. She also helps to coordinate an annual statewide self-advocacy conference, gives presentations on issues related to self-advocacy, and helps individuals advocate for themselves (e.g., accompanying them to meetings).

Angela is a young woman who worked for her state's self-determination project for about 2 years. After this, she decided to take a paid position 20 hours a week as coordinator for the state self-advocacy organization. In this role, she helped organize and support local self-advocacy groups, organized an annual statewide conference, and participated in trainings for providers and other groups of people (e.g., a training for independent support brokers, Protection and Advocacy). She also represented the state self-advocacy association in forging coalitions with other organizations, such as the State Council on Independent Living.

Special Initiatives or Projects   In recent years, when special systems change projects have been initiated, some of these have been designed to include self-advocates in central roles. A prime example was the Robert Wood Johnson Foundation self-determination grants that went to 19 states, which served to 1) involve people with developmental disabilities in designing and implementing systems change and 2) create systems change that would promote increased control and choice for people with developmental disabilities (Bradley et al., 2001; Moseley, 2001). For instance, in Vermont, the central work of the self-determination project was accomplished by four teams. Each team was composed of one parent, one service provider representative, and one self-advocate. Cindy first came into contact with the self-determination project because she and her mother were seeking more flexible support services for Cindy. After several months of working with the project team, Cindy was invited to speak about her experience working with the team. Over time, Cindy became more interested in speaking about her own experiences and working to help others gain more control and choice in their lives. She applied for and was offered a position working with the self-determination project. In this role, she worked with a team assisting individuals and families working on self-determination, giving presentations and trainings to various groups and organizations, and, in general, advocating for systems change to promote self-determination.

University Research Projects and Centers   There are still few but gradually increasing opportunities for self-advocates to be part of federal, state, and other types of research grants and projects (NCDDR, 2003). Since 1983, Doug has worked at the Center on Human Policy at Syracuse University as a self-advocacy coordinator. This work has been funded through various grants to the Center on Human Policy, some specifically focused on self-advocacy, and others focused more broadly on community integration and inclusion. As part of this role, he has worked locally and regionally to do individual advocacy, to do training about self-advocacy, and to help support and develop self-advocacy organizations. He has worked within the state to help support statewide self-advocacy networks and conduct trainings on systems change. At the national level, he has given many presentations and written numerous articles that address strategies for self-advocacy and systems change.

National Organizations   Over time, Hannah realized she wanted to do more advocacy work, and not just as a volunteer. As she got more involved, she said, "It was harder to squeeze it in as volunteer work in addition to my job." Her family was nervous about her making this change, as they were not sure she would find a paid job. Close friends who she had met through her involvement in self-advocacy supported her in her pursuit of advocacy work. At first, she found a paid position for one day a week working on criminal justice and disability issues as part of a grant. She did this for about a year, but realized that she really wanted to find full-time work. Through networking at a conference in 1996, Hannah was offered a full-time job with a state department of mental retardation; this job involved work on quality assurance, self-determination, and staff training. She stayed at this job for 3 years, and gained some valuable work experience. In January 2000, she decided she wanted a change and began looking for another job. She was hired by a national disability organization. She conducts training and presents at conferences relating to issues such as self-advocacy, self-determination, inclusion on boards and committees, employment, and other issues. She feels that this organization was thoughtful about why they wanted to hire a self-advocate, and what her role would be; in addition, she has determined the type of support she needs.

In addition to her job, Hannah continues with other volunteer connections, including the state developmental disabilities council, and the state self-advocacy group. Overall, it means a lot to her that she has full-time work involving advocating for and improving the lives of people with disabilities, as she feels it is crucial that people with disabilities play a role in these issues at all levels.

Having opportunities for paid advocacy and systems change work is very important to the individuals who were part of this study. At the same time, while this chapter focuses on paid work, it does not address the important aspect of volunteer self-advocacy work and activism for systems change, which are also critically important for these individuals. All of the people interviewed do self-advocacy on a volunteer basis, in addition to their paid work. They volunteer for self-advocacy organizations and advocate on behalf of people with disabilities in the context of a wide variety of local and state committees, organizations, and initiatives (e.g., human service agency boards, state committees, local transportation and human rights committees, criminal justice projects). Many also engage in various forms of social activism, including demonstrations. This volunteer work and activism allows them to advocate in ways that are not always possible through paid work.

CHALLENGES TO PAID SELF-ADVOCACY
AND SYSTEMS CHANGE WORK

The people we interviewed spoke of many different positive aspects of doing self-advocacy and systems change work. These include the opportunity to have a paid job that involves work that one is most passionate about, as well as having a sense that one's work is making a real change in the world that is having a beneficial impact on people's lives. At the same time, there are many challenges to doing self-advocacy and systems change work as part- or full-time paid employment.

Limited Leadership Positions

There are still very limited leadership opportunities for self-advocates, particularly those involving paid employment (Lakin & Turnbull, 2005; Powers et al., 2001; SABE, 2004). Self-advocacy organizations generally do not have adequate financial resources to pay staff and/or to do fundraising that would enable them to pay staff. Organizations that do pay staff often do so with funding from other organizations and these are generally part-time positions of 20 hours per week or less with no benefits. While funding from other organizations can be beneficial, it also can be a constraint to advocacy regarding systems issues. Other disability-related organizations are increasingly hiring individuals to work in a paid self-advocacy positions; however, research has found that the roles of self-advocates in such organizations are still quite limited (Bradley et al., 2001; Powers et al., 2001).

Inadequate Support

Self-advocates still experience difficulties in getting the amount or kind of support they need to do their job. Some self-advocacy positions have paid support workers built in. However, even with this, self-advocates have experienced difficulties (Lakin & Turnbull, 2005). For instance, among the self-advocates interviewed for this chapter, one person said that, "I feel like I'm interrupting the person from other work when I ask for something." Another characterized her support worker as "controlling." A third person talked about having to miss meetings that were part of her job due to lack of transportation. In addition, people talked about having to participate in meetings with co-workers who use jargon and other language that is inaccessible to them, without any explanation or assistance provided. One person commented, "I don't need it to be perfect, but I would like to have some understanding of what is going on."

Slow and Frustrating Pace of Change

The service system as a whole is still very bureaucratic, and many professionals and organizations that are part of this system are still reluctant to give up power and really listen to and collaborate with self-advocates.

Risks Associated With Self-Advocacy Work

By its nature, advocacy involves pushing and challenging people and systems to change. This work can lead to confrontation and conflict. This is sometimes threatening to self-advocates who still rely on the service system for supports that are crucial to their lives.

Financial Constraints

In paid positions, some people still have to be cautious about how much they earn so that their Medicaid benefits are not cut. One person who was interviewed had to relinquish his paid self-advocacy job because of benefits issues. Efforts to address this issue are being made nationally through implementation of the Ticket to Work and Work Incentive Program (Lakin & Turnbull, 2005).

Limitations to Advocacy

It is important to work for change both from within the system and beyond. At the same time, for self-advocates who have positions within the system, there are some limitations to the extent to which they can push for systems change from within.

Unsatisfactory Roles in Paid Positions

Due to the lack of self-advocates in leadership positions, and the scarcity of paid positions, self-advocates still sometimes feel isolated in paid positions. In addition, when they are working for other organizations (e.g., beyond self-advocacy organizations), they sometimes sense their role is a "token self-advocate role," or that their role and contribution has not been well thought out. Lack of proper supports can exacerbate feelings of isolation. Finally, people sometimes experience a sense of isolation based upon lack of true collaboration with others at a workplace or within an organization.

Despite the numerous challenges that exist, the positives far outweigh the negatives, and increasing numbers of self-advocates are seeking paid self-advocacy work. Having the support and collaboration of colleagues contributes significantly to diminishing the challenges. The following section discusses issues related to collaboration with self-advocates.

WHAT OTHERS CAN DO TO PROMOTE MEANINGFUL COLLABORATION WITH SELF-ADVOCATES

The work of self-advocates to promote systems change is sometimes strengthened by involvement and collaboration with others who are working for systems change. Increasingly, disability organizations and entities are, at least in theory, embracing the ideas of self-advocacy and self-determination. In practice, this entails an obligation to go beyond just giving self-advocates a place at the table; it involves promoting meaningful participation and inclusion of self-advocates. As called for by self-advocates, this requires real roles, not token roles, and true collaboration; and support for self-advocates and self-advocacy organizations. Efforts have and are being made in these directions, and lessons are being learned from these experiences.

Meaningful Roles and True Collaboration

For self-advocates, it is important that they now are beginning to have a place at the table concerning design and development of support services and other systems issues. At the same time, experience has shown that there are often still shortcomings in meaningful roles for and true collaboration with self-advocates (Bradley et al., 2001; Powers et al., 2001). For example, self-advocates who were interviewed indicated that when working with others, they still sometimes feel unclear about their role, feel that their role is a token role, and, in general, feel a lack of true partnership with colleagues.

Implementation of the state self-determination projects was a notable example of initiatives designed with self-advocates as core, central partici-pants. While there was significant variation between states and some short-comings in perhaps all of them, the aim was not only to create systems change so that self-advocates would have more choice and control, but that self-advocates would be centrally involved in creating this systems change. As one example, the experience of the Vermont Self-Determination Project illustrates strategies and lessons in this type of collaboration (Walker, Harris, Hall, Smith, & Shoultz, 2000).

The work of the project was organized based on teams of three people, with each team having three members or facilitators—including one person who represented service providers, a parent, and a self-advocate (i.e., consumer facilitator). As project team members worked to change the system in Vermont, they recognized that the way they worked together as a team and the lessons they learned from this were equally as important as the systems change that was accomplished. The project is as much about who it is that they are together, and how they accomplish things, as it is about what they go out and do.

There were four key factors (Walker et al., 2000) that contributed to create an atmosphere of collaboration:

1. *Commitment that all members of the team would have an active and meaningful role in all team activities.* At different times, team members played different roles, based upon interests, strengths, and experiences. However, it was clear that everyone had a role.

2. *Commitment to respecting one another and working to change preconceived notions.* It was important that team members recognized and acknowl-edged their preconceived notions and were willing to learn from one another.

3. *Commitment to open communication.* It was important that team members be attentive to the quality of their communication with one another and work

to address problems. This meant things such as giving each person a chance to speak, listening, and respecting differences of opinion.

4. *Commitment to support consumer participation.* Critical to successful collaboration was the commitment to fully support consumer participation, with flexibility in strategies and resources. This is discussed further in the next section.

While these factors did not ensure that self-advocates would always feel that their roles were meaningful or that team members would always work together smoothly and cohesively, they did create a framework for collaboration and for addressing problems with collaboration as they arose.

Support for Self-Advocates

As previously noted, in the past several years, increasing numbers of groups and organizations are seeking ways to collaborate with self-advocates, including through paid employment (Lakin & Turnbull, 2005). Support can be a key factor in the participation, and quality of participation, of people with disabilities in organizations, committees, and other groups. While most of these organizations are making attempts to provide support for the self-advocates who are working with them, there are still many shortcomings (Lakin & Turnbull, 2005). The self-advocates interviewed for this chapter report that often significant problems and deficiencies remain with the support they receive. For example, one self-advocate who has worked in numerous volunteer and paid positions commented, "It's been hard getting the right kind of support." In her current job, she has a full-time support person. But, in a past position, the person who supported her also had other simultaneous roles. She reflected, "I would always have to go looking for her and ask for help. I always felt like I was interrupting." Other self-advocates talked about the lack of predictable availability of a person to assist them with various job tasks, and about the lack of adequate support to help them understand written materials as well as to understand everything that was being discussed in meetings.

It is crucial that supports be individually designed based upon the person's needs and desires. This entails listening to and learning from self-advocates in order to determine the most effective supports. The Vermont Self-Determination Project provides an example of support that enabled self-advocates to be active co-workers and team members (Walker et al., 2000). On the teams, it was recognized that support of consumer facilitators was integral to the overall functioning of the teams as a whole. From the start, the project wanted to ensure that there was sufficient, quality support for consumer team members. Funding was provided so that each consumer facilitator could have a job coach. These people were hired individually, by each consumer facilitator, through a service agency of the person's choice. In addition, soon after the project was started, they identified the need for a project staff person who provided additional support to the consumer facilitators, and support to the teams as a whole. In terms of the relationships of other team members to the consumer facilitator, the vision of the project included the idea that team members could relate to each other as peers, and that the two nondisabled team members would not be in the position of having to provide support for the consumer team member.

There were a number of lessons learned about support for self-advocates from this team model of collaboration.

1. *It takes ongoing work to provide quality support for consumers.* For example, some of the consumers experienced frequent turnover of job coaches, which demanded attention from the consumer and team as a whole. In addition, it took ongoing work to figure out transportation, accessibility, and other logistics.

2. *It takes flexibility to provide quality support for consumers.* As noted above, after a few months of project work, it became clear that there was a need for another project staff person to provide additional support to the consumers and the teams as a whole. It was critical that the project had the flexibility to notice and respond to this need.

3. *While the project established guidelines about relationships between team members, these were not hard and fast rules.* It was important that there were guidelines intended to foster equitable roles for all team members and to prevent the consumer facilitators from having to depend on other team members for support. However, the real experience working together was not as clear cut as this. Sometimes when the consumer facilitator was without support, other team members stepped in to help out. At other times, when the consumer facilitator was having difficulties in his or her own life, team members offered suggestions and advice. While teammates without disabilities struggled with when or whether to offer advice, they did so based upon mutual, caring relationships that had evolved out of working together on a team. At the same time, consumer facilitators learned to set boundaries with their teammates as to when and where they wanted advice or assistance.

Effective collaboration with self-advocates necessitates central, meaningful roles for self-advocates and individualized support for participation. The experience of the Vermont Self-Determination Project reveals that ongoing effort and flexibility may be required to achieve such collaboration and that all who participate (not just the self-advocates) benefit from the collaboration.

CONCLUSION

Dybwad and Bersani commented on how people with developmental disabilities have come from being perceived as "feebleminded patients to empowered agents"(1996, p. 16). As part of this evolution of empowerment, self-advocates are increasingly finding opportunities for paid self-advocacy and systems change work. Nancy Ward reflected that in her early days of self-advocacy leadership, there were no role models (Ward & Shoultz, 2000). Today, there are many more role models and opportunities for self-advocates to move into leadership positions, including those involving paid work. Self-advocacy organizations are developing the capacity to hire paid staff. Also, an increasing number and variety of other organizations are seeking self-advocates to work with them. And, more often than in the past, this entails, in part, paid employment. Self-advocates and self-advocacy groups also are increasingly collaborating on local, state, and national levels with other disability and nondisability entities and organizations in doing advocacy work that contributes to significant change in service system practice and policy (Bradley et al., 2001; Lakin & Turnbull, 2005).

While opportunities for paid employment have increased, they are still limited. A future challenge includes greater expansion of the opportunities for self-advocates to be in leadership positions, including those that are paid, with adequate, individualized supports. Self-advocates in leadership positions still face the challenge of feeling isolated. This is exacerbated due to improper or inadequate supports for their positions. With this isolation comes a fear among some self-advocates of speaking up, lest they jeopardize relationships with agencies on whom they rely for support.

Today, self-advocates and their allies are calling for more leadership training opportunities that help them develop the skills and competencies to pursue a diverse range of leadership positions. Efforts are being undertaken to increase and expand the leadership opportunities for self-advocates (Powers et al., 2002). Self-advocates are at the forefront of these efforts at the state and national level. For example, at the state level in Oregon, self-advocates have formed Self-Advocates as Leaders (SAAL), an organization of self-advocates interested in developing leadership skills and becoming equal partners in policy and legislation that affects our lives. At the national level, SABE's Project Leadership has provided extensive training and information to self-advocates, parents, policymakers, and many others.

While there are many positive aspects to the entry of self-advocates into paid positions, there are also limitations to the advocacy that one can do within some of these positions. It is for this reason that many self-advocates in paid positions also continue to do volunteer advocacy work as well. And, it is a reason why self-advocates seek leadership positions within community organizations, committees, and boards, as well as paid employment.

One of Nancy Ward's visions is that self-advocates will one day "put ourselves out of business," and there will be true inclusion and thus, no need for such advocacy work (Ward & Shoultz, 2000, p. 181). However, it is clear that there remains much work to be done, with a critical need for involvement of self-advocates (Williams, 1994). It is important for self-advocates to be involved from many angles, both paid and volunteer, working within self-advocacy organizations and within or in collaboration with other organizations and initiatives. It is also very clear that self-advocates have tremendous commitment to self-advocacy and systems change work, whether paid or volunteer; it is much more than just work, but a life commitment and passion. All of those who were interviewed expressed that they had been doing advocacy, in one way another or, for much of their lives, and would continue to do so as long as necessary.

REFERENCES

Administration for Children and Families. (2004). *A charge we have to keep: Road map to success.* Washington, DC: President's Committee for People with Intellectual Disabilities, U.S. Department of Health and Human Services.

Bradley, V., Agosta, J., Smith, G., Taub, S., Ashbaugh, J., Silver, J., et al. (2001). *The Robert Wood Johnson Foundation Self-Determination Initiative: Final Impact Assessment Report.* Cambridge, MA: Human Services Research Institute.

Developmental Disabilities Assistance and Bill of Rights Act of 1975, PL 94-103, 100 Stat. 840, 42 U.S.C. §§ 6000 *et seq.*

Dybwad, G., & Bersani, H., Jr. (Eds.) (1996). *New voices: Self-advocacy by people with disabilities.* Cambridge, MA: Brookline Books.

Human Services Research Institute. (n.d.). *How your organization can sponsor self-advocates as AmeriCorps/VISTA members.* Portland, OR: Human Services Research Institute.

Lakin, K.C., & Turnbull, A. (2005). Self-advocacy, self-determination, and social freedom and opportunity. In K.C. Lakin & A. Turnbull (Eds.), *National goals and research for people with intellectual and developmental disabilities.* Baltimore: Paul H. Brookes Publishing Co.

Moseley, C. (2001). *Self-determination for persons with developmental disabilities: Final and summative program report.* Durham: University of New Hampshire Institute on Disability.

National Association of Councils on Developmental Disabilities. (2005). Councils support a diverse array of self-advocacy organizations. *Council Chronicles, 2*(1).

National Center for the Dissemination of Disability Research. (2003). Interview with Tia Nelis, self-advocate. *Research Exchange, 8*(3).

Powers, L.E., Ward, N., Ferris, L., Nelis, T., Ward, M., Wieck, C., et al. (2002). Leadership by people with disabilities in self-determination systems change. *Journal of Disability Policy Studies, 13*(2), 125–133.

Self Advocates Becoming Empowered (SABE). (2004, Spring). Self-advocates as leaders. *SABE Newsletter.* Retrieved January 16, 2007, from http://www.asksaal.org

Shoultz, B., & Ward, N. (1996). Self Advocates Becoming Empowered: The birth of a national organization in the U.S. In G. Dybwad & H. Bersani, Jr. (Eds.), *New voices: Self-advocacy by people with disabilities* (pp. 216–234). Cambridge, MA: Brookline Books.

Walker, P., Harris, P., Hall, M., Smith, V., & Shoultz, B. (2000). *Self-determination in Vermont: Contributions of the Vermont Self-Determination Project.* Syracuse, NY: Center on Human Policy.

Ward, N., & Shoultz, B. (2000). My leadership career. In R. Traustadottir & K. Johnson (Eds.), *Women with intellectual disabilities: Finding a place in the world* (pp. 172–181). London: Jessica Kingsley Publishers.

Whittico, P., & Ingram, T. (1994). The history and accomplishments of self-advocates becoming empowered. *IMPACT: Feature Issue on Self-Advocacy, 7*(1), 2–3.

Williams, B. (1994). Self-advocates and advocates: Voices for continued change. *IMPACT: Feature Issue on Self-Advocacy, 7*(1), 13.

CHAPTER SEVEN

Promoting a Good Old Age

Strategies for Identifying Interests and Developing Community Connections

JENNIE TODD, JANE HARLAN-SIMMONS, AND PAMELA M. WALKER

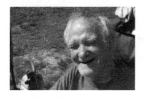

Many older people today enjoy very active and engaged lives. After pursuing fulfilling careers, many people look forward to retirement and increased time with family and friends, as well as increased time to travel and to pursue hobbies and interests or develop new ones. According to Rowe and Khan,

Most older people in the general population make productive contributions of some kind, more in the form of informal help giving and unpaid volunteer work than paid employment. Among people 55 years of age and older, more than 9 out of 10 do housework; 8 out of 10 do home maintenance; 7 out of 10 provide help of various kinds to friends and relatives; and more than 3 out of 10 work as volunteers in churches, hospitals, and other organizations. Almost as many older people work for pay as volunteer, about 3 out of 10. Only 2% report no productive activity whatsoever. (1998, p. 170)

People with disabilities want the same things we all do in old age. A "good old age" includes physical health, material security, supportive networks of family and friends, pursuit of meaningful work, and other interests and hobbies (Hawkins, 1999). Yet, options for aging adults with developmental disabilities approaching and surpassing retirement age are still limited, and many aging people are served in segregated day services settings. There are few options for retirement within the developmental disability services system (Heller, 2000). Older people with disabilities are sometimes reluctant to retire or discontinue participation at a sheltered workshop or day habilitation center, fearful that it will mean loss of income, loss of social connections outside their home, and being forced into a nursing home if they no longer attend day service settings (Heller, 1999). When they do participate in community activities, these are often based on a congregate approach such as group outings, volunteering as a group, and the like (Kultgen, Harlan-Simmons, & Todd, 2000). Without concerted effort and ongoing support from staff and families, and cross-system collaboration, aging people with disabilities are not afforded opportunities to be contributing community members nor provided some of the lifestyle choices that promote successful aging.

One approach that can enhance the lives of people with disabilities, including those who are older, is increased opportunities to develop and pursue interests and community connections (Amado, 1993; Harlan, Todd, & Holz, 1998). This chapter focuses on strategies to promote meaningful daytimes for older adults with developmental disabilities. The primary emphasis of the chapter is on strategies for community building, based on individual interests. The chapter begins with a presentation of efforts at the Indiana Institute on Disability and Community to assist older people with disabilities to identify and pursue interests. The second part of the chapter describes technical assistance with community building provided to agency staff by the Institute on Disability and Community. Even with significant effort directed toward identification of interests and establishment of community connections, opportunities to be part of the community can vary tremendously based on the context of day and residential support services provided to a given individual. The chapter concludes with discussion of systems issues that can facilitate or impede community involvement for older citizens with disabilities.

IDENTIFICATION AND PURSUIT OF
INTERESTS: ROUNDTABLE APPROACH

Researchers at the Indiana Institute on Disability and Community's Center on Aging and Community (CAC) in Bloomington, Indiana wanted to know what aging people with developmental disabilities saw as the key issues in their lives and what they thought was vital to promote a healthy transition toward later life. In 1994, CAC established an advisory board of 10 older adults with developmental disabilities from a four county area to help figure this out. The criteria for board participation were a yearlong monthly commitment and representation of both themselves and other voices not in attendance.

One of the earliest topics the advisory board discussed was retirement. When members were asked what retirement meant to them, responses ranged from moving to Florida to quitting the sheltered workshop and getting a job in the community. Most wanted to visit family, take trips, and enjoy leisure activities. There were misconceptions about retirement and a lack of accurate and available information on the subject. For example, some people thought that retirement meant they would have to move to a nursing home. Equally notable through the discussion was the scarcity of interests, hobbies, and relationships never developed or nurtured throughout their lifetime.

Based upon this feedback, researchers at CAC submitted a successful grant proposal to the U.S. Administration on Developmental Disabilities for a 5-year project. The overarching goal of the grant was the facilitation of roundtable discussions coupled with staff technical assistance on community building methodologies with groups from six different Indiana human service agencies, which will be fully described later in the chapter. Two of the authors of this chapter (Todd & Harlan-Simmons) served as two of the facilitators and consultants providing technical assistance for the project.

The notion of roundtable discussions resulted from the experiences and time with the original CAC Advisory Board. To locate agencies interested in being sites for roundtable facilitation and staff technical assistance on community building methodologies, CAC sent broad-based announcements to Indiana day service providers. In agency selection, expectations such as commitment to the success of the project, manpower, and follow through were discussed to help carefully choose the six sites.

Roundtable discussions gave participants a voice while providing agency staff information to better design services and supports. The structure and content of roundtable discussions helps people discover their interests and priorities while crafting a vision and action plan. All strategies were designed to achieve more person-centered services and provide opportunities for new opportunities and relationships.

Roundtables were designed as a forum for discussion of an array of issues with a focus on self-determination and aging issues and including ongoing or current personal struggles facing the members. Roundtable work was designed to offer a safe venue for discussion facilitated by CAC staff with no agenda except the focus mentioned above. The researchers were there to facilitate, record, and provide corresponding materials and activities complementing the groups' chosen topics. Issues previously identified by the CAC Advisory Board and others were roles, rights and responsibilities, life transitions, and group home de-certifications.

Roundtable meetings were geared toward persons age 50 and older, but open to any person using the agency's services and wanting to attend. At two sites only people with disabilities attended the roundtable discussions while at two other sites staff were invited to join, as some members needed more intensive assistance with communication and mobility for hands-on activities. However, staff were asked to take a supportive role only. Meetings were held every 3–4 weeks, with the expectation that it would take several months to develop the rapport with the group necessary for full participation and open discussion. Roundtable meetings were generally scheduled for 1½ hours on average.

Each member of the roundtable was given a personalized three-ring binder notebook at the second meeting. Notebooks were designed to be both person specific, intended to record their dreams and preferences, as well as group specific, intended to record ideas generated by the group as a whole. The intent of the notebook was to provide a place for all roundtable information to be stored, reviewed, and shared with others.

The focus of roundtable activities was for participants to identify and clarify interests, dreams, and visions of the future. In addition, roundtable members discussed choices and control in their lives, and the barriers to achieving their goals and dreams. Most members had little experience dreaming about their futures and this seemed to be unexplored territory. Some participants had difficulty summoning sufficient hope and vision to dream about the future. Members who allowed themselves to dream tended to then rule the dream out based on lack of money. Often, dreams focused on low-level employment (e.g., mowing lawns, sweeping and cleaning in fast food restaurants) or ordinary life experiences (e.g., seeing family, going to a movie, traveling to a nearby city, going on a date, getting a job, eating out, getting a cat). Occasionally, people articulated bigger dreams, such as buying an accessible vehicle, becoming a police officer, or owning a home. Sometimes dreams emerged unexpectedly as other topics were addressed. A videotape depicting the social life of an active, independent man became the catalyst for a roundtable member to express her fervent wish to move out of a group home, where she felt she did not belong, into an apartment with her boyfriend. Deeply held desires could sometimes be intuited from members' nonverbal reactions. While viewing a videotape, a woman who didn't speak became very excited when she saw a young woman with a communication device that she could program to say what she wanted using a synthesized voice.

Following the identification of dreams, group members discussed the barriers to the pursuit of these dreams. They mentioned things like transportation, limitations on choice-making imposed by family members and/or staff, people who did not believe in them, and lack of self-initiative. Solutions along with next steps were brainstormed and discussed for each posed barrier within the context of a specific individual, providing some problem-solving experience.

Challenges to Successful Roundtable Work

A challenge to successful roundtable work is the lack of follow-up by support staff. Roundtable discussions inspired and motivated the group but agency or residential providers soon squelched those feelings by discounting or ignoring preferences.The providers often did not have resources or creative strategies to follow through on many ideas or suggestions. The concern was that roundtable members were more confused and frustrated.

As part of technical support, CAC researchers worked with each roundtable member and their agency support staff to develop a personal profile of interests, as well as possible community places and activities, while spelling out action steps toward community involvement. Later, researchers facilitated a follow-up session with staff to discuss progress. In reality, nothing changed for most people. Roundtable work was successful while researchers were available to facilitate the discussions. However, once staff were on their own, staff members often got caught up in other responsibilities. The roundtable work and follow-up were not high priorities and often fell by the wayside.

SUPPORTING AGENCY STAFF AS COMMUNITY BUILDERS: STRATEGIES FOR CREATIVE PLANNING WITH OLDER ADULTS

This section of the chapter describes the community building assistance that was provided to agencies during the community building process. This was a one-to-one approach focusing on discovering a person's interests and desires, while strategizing to develop meaningful community roles and relationships. The approach was discussed as a tool for achieving a desirable retirement. All stories describe people approaching or surpassing retirement age. All strategies were designed to achieve more person-centered services and provide opportunities for new experiences and relationships.

To complement the roundtable work, agency staff were immersed in the tools and techniques of community building. The objective was to give staff the skills and support to connect roundtable participants in meaningful ways to their community and for roundtable members to see progress made toward their dreams. The community building process, based on the concept of person-centered planning (e.g., Mount, 1992; O'Brien & O'Brien, 1998), has been described in *A Guide to Building Community Membership* (Harlan et al., 1998) as progressing through stages in which a person begins exploring their community to find their niche for participation and contribution. The stages are not always distinct nor are they predictably sequential. The process is fluid and flexible. Three stages are described below: discovering a person's interests and desires; promoting meaningful community participation; and cultivating relationships.

Discovery of a Person's Interests and Desires

The process of discovery of a person's interests and desires can be applied to people of all ages. In this chapter it is considered in relation to older adults. Some older adults who have lived in congregate settings for most or all of their lives may have had little opportunity to explore individual interests. Others may need to reexamine interests following major life changes (e.g., changes in physical capacity, movement to a new home, loss of family or friends). In order to best assist an individual with community participation, staff who are community builders need to know the person well, based in part upon time spent together in the community. The initial phase of getting to know a person outside of their agency setting may necessitate exploring a wide variety of places and activities over several months. This investigation cannot be done as part of a group. When the person is allowed to seek out new places and try new activities with one-on-one support, he or she can be a full participant in determining the direction that the exploration will take. Getting to know the person also requires one-to-one time because people react to environments differently when not in a group. Community members will be less likely to invoke expectations bred by stereotypes, and more likely to engage in social interaction, if the person isn't surrounded by others who are together solely because of a shared label and a staff shortage.

Listening and watching carefully for body language and other cues from the person will lay the groundwork for identifying successful places and roles in the community later on. It is not necessary for people to communicate verbally in order to get to know their passions and talents.

Vern was looking for volunteer work in the community. His community builder and anyone else who knew Vern were aware he was a major sports fan. The community builder planned to look for volunteer opportunities relating to sports. Wanting to discover other sides of Vern, the community builder took him to an art museum. Although Vern's communication might be perceived as limited to movements signaling a yes or no response, she could immediately sense his excitement there, particularly at the portrait paintings and glass sculptures. After the revelation in the museum, Vern and his community builder decided to find an art class for him. When an interest becomes apparent, new activities suggest themselves. Trying those activities, in turn, provides more information about the best way to proceed.

Getting to know someone in a new setting can create fresh possibilities for those who have been labeled a behavior problem. Problems (e.g., antisocial behavior, aggression, actions that are harmful to oneself or others) can disappear if the customary environment is replaced by one in which the person flourishes, and if people with negative expectations are replaced with people who have shared interests and positive expectations. The person is starting with a clean slate.

At her day program facility, and sometimes at the group home, Frieda would curse, mutter, make angry gestures, and keep to herself. When her community builder took her to an all-ages country line dancing place, Frieda was transformed. She blended in with the crowd and became absorbed in moving to the music. When she felt like a break, she bought herself a soda at the refreshment counter. The behaviors she had accumulated over many years in institutional settings were absent.

It is instantly recognizable when the person has found something they love to do, something that brings out their best. These are the clues that make possible the visioning process that comprises the next stage of community building.

Promoting Meaningful Community Participation

Having built a foundation of information and experience during the phase of learning and exploration, it is now possible to create a vision of how and where the older person will emerge into the place of opportunity, exchange, and connection associated with the notion of community. Where feasible, person-centered planning tools such as Planning Alternative Tomorrows with Hope (PATH; Pearpoint, O'Brien, & Forest, 1992) or personal futures planning (Mount, 1992) can effectively incorporate a vision for community participation. Convening a group of people, including those who have known the person for years as well as those who have no preconceptions about the person, makes the outcomes of planning richer and takes the burden off the community builder. The vision is a shared image of the person's identified gifts, preferences, and wishes, and the roles and places in which those gifts will unfold and develop. How and where can the person truly be himself or herself while contributing to the larger community? What keys does he or she hold that will open the door to the give-and-take of relationships with fellow citizens, to freely given companionship?

In this phase of establishing community connections, the vision for community participation takes tangible shape as gifts, preferred activities, and environments are matched with the specific assets of the locale. The community builder uses resources such as newspapers, telephone directories, Internet listings, community calendars, the chamber of commerce, and reference librarians to seek out relevant associations, organizations, churches, or businesses. The riches of personal networks can be mined to find "bridge builders" who are active in a particular group. Bridge builders are outgoing people who seem to know everyone, who have some status in the group, and can introduce the newcomer to others who share his or her interests.

The community builder seeks out sites that are a good match for the individual's habits and inclinations; sites that come as close as possible to the envisioned ideal. The task is to find welcoming places, where there are people with whom to socialize and where there is a good chance of developing something meaningful for the person to do. A site can be as informal as a neighborhood tavern, a small-town beauty parlor, or a horse stable. It might be an urban art center, a busy truck repair business, a YMCA, a radio station, or a quiet church office. It is a place where the person smiles and sparkles.

Without speaking, Kevin showed a strong preference for working with paper and liked to carry a briefcase. He kept his distance from the others in his day program, gravitating towards people who weren't labeled with a disability. His community builder took her cues from his interests and helped him get to know many of the business proprietors within the area of a few blocks downtown. She knew the small city where they both lived and was comfortable chatting with long-time residents. Kevin was initially very hesitant, but became more comfortable as they regularly visited various businesses to say hello, and found small jobs involving paper that he could do to help out. They spent time at the counter of the corner coffee shop and he became well liked by the proprietor. Kevin's activities did not require transportation, facilitating ongoing participation independent of the community builder. He spent time at the businesses on a regular basis so that the people he met there had a chance to get to know him. His role could be characterized as "Mr. Main Street."

Cultivating Relationships

Once regular participation at a site is underway, the individual and his or her community builder can begin to look for promising relationships to encourage and nurture. Cultivating relationships requires both delicacy and persistence. The community builder can creatively support the focus person to make him or her known and appreciated by bringing bagels, donuts, or a bouquet of flowers, sending cards for birthdays and holidays, or asking others to go out for a soda or coffee. The community builder can help the focus person practice making conversation, for example, by role playing a scenario of asking others about their weekends, inquiring about spouses or children, and so forth. A person who doesn't communicate verbally can be assisted to bring in items to share, such as photos or memorabilia, in order to help others to get to know him or her. A powerful catalyst for the formation of closer ties is to bring a person into the sphere of community members who share at least one of his or her interests.

David, an avid euchre player, reserves part of every Tuesday for playing cards with other seniors at the community center. They save him a seat because he is a good euchre player, but also because they find him a pleasant, caring, and fun person to be around. With David's sense of humor and love of horses, it wasn't long before an invitation was extended to join a Saturday trip to the horse track.

For older persons, the reactivation of dormant relationships from the past can be meaningful and satisfying, offering opportunities for reminiscing and affirming a sense of continuity.

Trudy became a regular visitor at a nursing facility where she found old friends to talk to, including her very elderly former schoolteacher. While at first she was anxious to keep the community builder nearby, the latter eventually disappeared for a period of time while Trudy happily conversed with the patients she knew.

Friends cannot be produced at will by the community builder. However, the broader the person's exposure to various acquaintances, the greater the likelihood that the chemistry of friendship will work. In other words, the more places of participation, the more opportunities to meet people; the more opportunities to meet people, the more chances to develop relationships; the more relationships, the greater the opportunity for friendships.

David, the man who loved playing euchre, also developed his interest in art by studying ceramics at a community art center. The ceramics teacher was impressed with the way David's hand built clay pieces inspired the other class members. She wanted to learn more about David's life outside the art class. A circle of support had been forming to help David move out of his group home, and the teacher began to attend his circle meetings. As this was only a six-week class, the intent had been for David to learn something new and do something he enjoyed. At minimum, an activity such as an art class can give an individual something to talk about; it can make him or her a more interesting person. The continuing relationship with the ceramics teacher was a lasting bonus!

Sooner or later the community builder must fade into the background to allow social connections to blossom. With thoughtful planning and use of natural supports, people who are usually at the site can provide assistance where necessary, and sometimes transportation as well. When a connection is successful, the relationship might extend beyond the activity or location where it took root.

Roger and his community builder had been frequenting a family-oriented franchise restaurant for breakfast each week. He got to know the waitresses and the manager, who would have some of his favorite fruit or cookies ready to bring with his coffee when he arrived. Roger and the manager were having conversations at each visit, and they discovered a common commitment to their Christian faith. Wishing to let the two develop their friendship independently of her, Roger's community builder decided to ask the manager if it would be okay for her to bring Roger to the restau-

rant and then come back after a time to pick him up. This was agreeable, and they had coffee without her the next week. The community builder reported that it had taken a long time to get to this point, but she felt her persistence was well rewarded. Later, at Roger's invitation, he and the restaurant manager began attending Bible study classes together.

SYSTEMS ISSUES: CONCLUSIONS AND RECOMMENDATIONS

As noted previously, opportunities for community building, and thus, for community membership, can be either significantly enhanced or hindered by the other services the individual receives, particularly residential services, as well as by the degree of collaboration between those who provide services. A few of the critical service system factors are outlined below.

Flexible, Individualized Day and Residential Services

Community opportunities are enhanced when day and residential services are community-based, individualized, and flexible, versus facility-based. Within traditional services, people with disabilities are often required to be out of their group home for a specific number of hours per day. They are often forced to move to more restrictive facilities or nursing homes when their support needs increased (Taylor, 1988). Older people may not want to or be able to leave their home for work and other day activities to the same extent as when they were younger. In addition, they may want to pursue involvement within new community contexts. Flexible day and residential services enable individuals with disabilities, including those who are older, to live in (or remain in) their own or shared homes in the community, and to increase the support within the home as people's support needs change, so that they can "age in place" (Janicki, 1999). Alternative day services, such as those provided through Neighbours, Inc., in New Jersey (as described in Chapter 5), give individuals who are older the opportunity to retire and stay home or pursue community interests, rather than continue working or attending day activities centers. Combined day and residential services funding, as utilized by Katahdin Friends, Inc., in Maine, offers the flexibility to support people in their own homes or within the community during the day.

Interface and Collaboration Between Day and Residential Service

Opportunities for community participation can be significantly enhanced by collaboration between day and residential service providers. For example, at the point when an individual is beginning regular participation at a community site, issues may arise in the interface between the community builder, when employed by a day services provider, and the agency that provides residential services for the individual. The support of residential staff is important in making sure the person is regularly prepared for attendance at his or her meeting, volunteer job, class, or other activity. Residential staff needs to be involved early on in the process so that they are informed of the purpose and value of the community building time, enlisted for their help, and kept abreast of progress and small successes. Good communication is essential to avoid sabotage (whether accidental or deliberate).

When Frieda went line dancing on Tuesday nights, the group home made sure she finished her supper on time and helped her to look her best. They took her shopping for a western-style shirt so she could look like one of the regulars. The community builder made sure she was on time to pick up and drop off Frieda. They shared stories about Frieda's enjoyment of the "Cowboy Stroll" and other dances.

Sometimes, however, creative circumvention of staff resistance and unnecessary regulations is necessary.

Larry is a Roman Catholic who lived in a group home where the only opportunity to worship was with the Protestant minister who visited the residence on Sundays. Judy, a day services staff member from another agency who was acting as Larry's community builder, was a practicing Catholic. She began taking Larry to Mass at a local church of his choosing. There was a church van that could pick him up, but Judy, who believed Larry was capable of traveling independently, had to ride along with him to assuage the concerns of the group home staff. Eventually she drove her car to the church to meet Larry, and he rode in the church van without her, unbeknownst to the staff. Once it was proved that he could do this without a problem, the staff offered no further objections.

Collaborative planning by day and residential services staff is also important to help ensure "aging in place" (Janicki, 1999). For instance, planning is required for individuals who live with aging parents, so they can prepare for the death of a parent or the need for changes in support and living situations. In addition, planning should encompass community participation, pursuit of interests, and social relationships. Adults should assume a central role in this process (Hawkins, 1999; Heller, 2000).

Finally, collaboration of day and residential services staff with aging services can help enhance opportunities for community membership for older adults with disabilities. Initiatives of this sort have been undertaken in a number of states (Hacker, McCallion, & Janicki, 2000; Sherman & Bloom, 2000). Local agencies on aging are a valuable resource for assistance for older adults. The Older Americans Act of 1965 (PL 89-73) funds a range of services for adults age 60 years and older, such as senior centers, nutrition sites, home-delivered meals, homemaker services, and transportation, among others. Such services could be critical to assisting an older individual with a disability to remain in the community. The Aging and Developmental Disabilities Interagency Effort in Florida was an example of such collaboration (Sherman & Bloom, 2000). For this collaboration it was essential to have support at the state administrative level, as well as at the local level.

Staff as Community Builders

Inadequate salaries and opportunities for advancement diminish the pool from which agencies can hire employees possessing the necessary qualities of good community builders. Staff who were accustomed to acting as caretakers or teachers were not always comfortable in the community builders' role. Some staff members whose jobs had changed from facility-based to community-based support had greater difficulty figuring out what to do outside the agency; had predetermined, negative notions about the focus person; and had difficulty letting go of their previous daily routine. Some made the transition well; however, they were usually the strongest members of the staff and were called in to handle crises or fill-in for needed billable hours.

CAC researchers found that much staff community building time was unfocused and nonspecific. Time was spent going to stores, restaurants, or movies without an overarching goal to discover the individual's interests, or to identify the individual's strengths and enthusiasms. In part, this may reflect a larger society's preoccupation with consumption and entertainment in the wake of a decline in civic participation and membership in social organizations (Putnam, 2000). In what came to be called the "Wal-Mart syndrome," staff had difficulty conceptualizing one-on-one time outside of the facility as an opportunity for developing a person's interests and creating lasting relationships. Rather, staff preferred assisting the older individual to accomplish errands and shopping. When asked, "Why Wal-Mart?" CAC researchers were commonly told, "He or she wanted to go there" or "We had your list but he chose Wal-Mart." The person's need to make active contributions and to belong to a group of people who share common interests was not easily recognized or respected.

Some agencies choose to hire one staff member or a few staff members for a specific community builder position. While this person can play a critical role within agencies, it is also important that all staff, to some degree, see community building as part of their role. To this end, agencies should design training and mentoring that helps staff develop their skills in community building and facilitating social relationships. At the same time, there are limits to the degree to which community building skills can be developed. In the end, there are also various personality traits that are unique to the tasks of community building. Prospective employees who are comfortable with people from all walks of life and with the unpredictable and unknown, and who are well-connected themselves, are good choices as community builders.

Agency Commitment

In addition to attracting and hiring skilled community builders, it is essential that there be agencywide commitment to efforts at community building. Though promotion of community involvement may be an essential piece of their mission statement, in reality, due to current funding streams and billable hour requirements, it often takes a back seat to all other services and supports. The best intended community builders are faced with the challenge of only having a certain number of hours per week to do one-to-one community work, with any agency crisis taking precedence. In this climate, it is important for agencies to revisit their mission so as not to lose sight of this aspect of the agency's mission.

To some extent, agencies must trust that staff are not using company time to conduct personal business in the name of community building. In addition, agencies are not accustomed to measuring or rewarding outcomes for pursuits not easily subsumed under vocational or habilitation goals. It is one thing to demonstrate that people are paying taxes on wages earned, or performing daily tasks with greater independence. It is more difficult to quantify the pride and satisfaction of a valued role, the sense of security and belonging in being part of a regularly attended group, the warmth of a freely-given relationship, and the excitement of having something to share that is truly one's own.

Furthermore, agencies may be hesitant to put consumers in situations where the agency might be held liable for their harm in an accident, crime situation, or other unforeseen circumstance. Ironically, few agencies recognize the harm they inflict by excluding people in the name of protection.

A sense of identity, an array of interests, and a network of relationships established throughout the years appear to be the essence of a satisfying older age. People who have been segregated for years are at greater risk of finding themselves lonely, isolated, and unproductive in their later years. The older adults we have worked with consistently communicated how much they value personal, freely-given relationships. Many of the adults expressed their feelings of loneliness and isolation. Not surprisingly, research among the general population demonstrates a strong link between social connections and well-being in the later years, membership in groups and organizations being a key variable (Rowe & Kahn, 1998.) If increasing opportunities for participation were not sufficiently valuable as an antidote to empty days and evenings and as a source of valued roles, such opportunities are also a goldmine of potential social connections.

One-to-one community building work has been discussed here as an avenue for providing adults approaching and of retirement age with more meaningful and satisfying pursuits and social relationships. Although person-centered approaches have gained ground through innovations in the areas of employment, transition planning, and housing, older adults with disabilities are frequently offered "cookie-cutter options" (e.g., group activities such as games or van rides may be offered without regard for each individual's interests and preferences), if any, for how and with whom they spend their time. In supporting service agency staff and administrators to accomplish this work in collaboration with those whom they serve, a number of challenges must be met. It was the authors' experience that, even in agencies where it is a stated mission to enrich and support the social networks and community participation of its constituency, the structures and policies necessary to accomplish this goal may be insufficient.

Targeted training and hands-on experience mentored by role models are needed in order to assist staff to master the tasks of collaborative exploration, creative strategizing, bridge-building, and facilitating. In addition, administrative support, flexible funding streams, recognition of leadership in the field, and other creative incentives need to be in place for long-term community building success.

This chapter described structured contexts in which service providers and policymakers can learn from the experts: Older persons with disabilities have a great deal to say and have some excellent ideas. Many are clear on what they want, which usually is no more—and often less—than the general public takes for granted. Support can be provided to enable this significant and growing segment of the population to experience the range of choices available in our communities. Older individuals can be empowered to identify and articulate their preferences, concerns, and priorities. It is possible to value and facilitate attainment of the dreams and goals of people who have been excluded from the rewards of retirement. By walking with and listening to those whose voices have not been heard, policies and services that promote fulfillment in the later years can be designed and implemented.

REFERENCES

Amado, A.N. (Ed.) (1993). *Friendships and community connections between people with and without developmental disabilities.* Baltimore: Paul H. Brookes Publishing Co.

Hacker, K.S., McCallion, P., & Janicki, M.P. (2000). Outreach and assistance using area agencies on aging. In M.P. Janicki & E.F. Ansello (Eds.), *Community supports for aging adults with lifelong disabilities* (pp. 439–456). Baltimore: Paul H. Brookes Publishing Co.

Harlan, J., Todd, J., & Holtz, P. (1998). *A guide to building community membership for older adults with disabilities.* Bloomington, IN: Institute for the Study of Developmental Disabilities.

Hawkins, B. (1999). Rights, place of residence, and retirement: Lessons from case studies on aging. In S.S. Herr & G. Weber (Eds.), *Aging, rights, and quality of life* (pp. 93–108). Baltimore: Paul H. Brookes Publishing Co.

Heller, T. (1999). Emerging models. In S.S. Herr & G. Weber (Eds.), *Aging, rights, and quality of life* (pp. 149–166). Baltimore: Paul H. Brookes Publishing Co.

Heller, T. (2000). Supporting adults with intellectual disabilities and their families in planning and advocacy: A literature review. In. J. Hammel & S.M. Nochajski (Eds.), *Aging and developmental disability: Current research, programming, and practice implications* (pp. 59–73). Binghamton, NY: The Haworth Press.

Janicki, M.P. (1999). Public policy and service design. In S.S. Herr & G. Weber (Eds.), *Aging, rights, and quality of life* (pp. 289–310). Baltimore: Paul H. Brookes Publishing Co.

Kultgen, P., Harlan-Simmons, J., & Todd, J. (2000). Community membership. In M.P. Janicki & E.F. Ansello (Eds.). *Community supports for aging adults with lifelong disabilities* (pp. 153–166). Baltimore: Paul H. Brookes Publishing Co.

Mount, B. (1992). *Person-centered planning: A sourcebook of values, ideas, and methods to encourage person-centered development.* New York: Graphic Futures.

O'Brien, J., & O'Brien, C.L. (Eds.). (1998). *A little book about person-centered planning.* Toronto: Inclusion Press.

Older Americans Act of 1965, PL 89-73, 42 U.S.C. §§ 3001 *et seq.*

Pearpoint, J., O'Brien, J., & Forest, M. (1992). *PATH.* Toronto: Inclusion Press.

Putnam, R. (2000). *Bowling alone: The collapse and revival of American community.* New York: Simon & Schuster.

Rowe, J.W., & Kahn, R.L. (1998). *Successful aging.* New York: Pantheon.

Sherman, J.M., & Bloom, P.A. (2000). Statewide organizational development. In M.P. Janicki & E.F. Ansello (Eds.), *Community supports for aging adults with lifelong disabilities* (pp. 493–507). Baltimore: Paul H. Brookes Publishing Co.

Taylor, S.J. (1988). Caught in the continuum: A critical analysis of the principle of the least restrictive environment. *Journal of The Association for Persons with Severe Handicaps, 13*(1), 45–53.

CHAPTER EIGHT

Moving from Facility-Based Day Services to Integrated Employment and Community Supports

PATRICIA ROGAN AND JEFFREY L. STRULLY

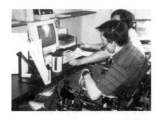

Despite more than 25 years and over 300,000 examples of people with disabilities working in integrated jobs through supported employment (Braddock, Rizzolo, & Hemp, 2004), the majority of federal and state funding for day services in the United States is directed to congregate, segregated facility-based programs (Braddock et al., 2004; Lawhead, 2005). Rusch and Braddock (2004) presented state mental retardation/developmental disability (MR/DD) data indicating that separate employment services receive four times more in financial resources than do integrated employment services. It is appalling to note that approximately 75% of individuals served in rehabilitation programs remain in sheltered workshops and day activity programs (Butterworth, Metzel, Boeltzig, Gilmore, & Sulweski, 2005; Wehman & Bricount, 1999). In fact, the number of people in facility-based programs has risen from 236,614 in 1988 to 365,165 in 2002 (Braddock et al., 2004).

The continuum of services, whereby people with disabilities are expected to earn their way into the community by getting ready in segregated settings, is alive and well (Taylor, 1988). A readiness mentality exists among service providers and others, resulting in the belief that people need to get ready for integrated employment and/or community access by spending time, often many years, in a segregated facility. Further exacerbating the situation is the fact that knowledge, skills, and resources related to supporting people with disabilities in meaningful daily routines is lacking among many service providers, despite the fact that a wealth of information is readily available in multiple formats.

Efforts to design rich and meaningful daytimes with and for people with significant disabilities rarely include segregated facilities if true choice and accompanying experiences are present. In other words, when individuals have had opportunities to experience integrated employment that is well matched to their interests, abilities, and needs, and when appropriate supports are in place, few choose segregated facilities (Murphy & Rogan, 1995; Murphy, Rogan, Hanley, Kincaid, & Royce-Davis, 2002). A recent study included interviews with 210 adults with intellectual disabilities in 19 sheltered workshops, their respective families or caregivers ($N = 185$), and staff members of these workshops ($N = 224$) (Migliore, Mank, Grossi, & Rogan, in press). Results indicated that the majority of respondents believed that adults with intellectual disabilities could work in the community if sufficient supports were provided, regardless of the severity of the disability. When service providers are entrenched in a facility-based mode of funding and service delivery, it is difficult to provide the individualized supports required of community-based services. Thus, supported employment opportunities may not be offered to individuals, or, if they are, they may not be of sufficient quality and scope to ensure customer satisfaction and success. Unfortunately, most community rehabilitation programs in the United States continue to offer segregated services as their primary mode of service delivery. Supported employment services have been added to the continuum of services, but a major shift from facility-based to community-based services has yet to occur on a national level (Butterworth et al., 2005). A mere 15% of organizations report downsizing their facilities (Wehman, Revell, & Kregel, 1998) and 80% of states do not consider downsizing a priority (Mank, Cioffi, & Yovanoff, 2003).

Research has shown that quality of life outcomes are better for those in supported employment compared to their counterparts in segregated day services (Gilmore & Butterworth, 1996; McCaughrin, Ellis, Rusch, & Heal, 1993; Wehman & Bricout, 1999). People are more integrated, earn more money, develop more skills, decrease their dependence on federal assistance, and increase their satisfaction and self-esteem as a result of integrated employment (Hernandez, Keys, & Balcazar, 2002; Kiernan & Schalock, 1997; Mank, 1994; Thompson, Powers, & Houchard, 1992; Wehman & Bricout, 1999).

In a study for the President's Task Force on the Employment of Adults with Disabilities, Rogan, Grossi, Mank, Haynes, & Thomas (2001) tracked the outcomes of former workshop participants who are now in supported employment. See Table 8.1 for a comparison of these outcomes.

Table 8.1. Comparison of outcomes of former workshop participants who are now in supported employment

	Sheltered workshop	Supported employment
Hours/Week	25	21
Wage/Hour	$2.30	$5.75
Wages/Month	$175.69	$455.97

Although it appears that people worked more hours in the sheltered facility than in supported employment, people did not work the entire time in the facility. Given the fact that there were periods of downtime when there was no work, and other activities were included in the day, such as music, counseling, and therapy sessions, the amount of actual work time was, in fact, less than those in supported employment.

Supported employment has proven to be more beneficial than facility-based programs for people with disabilities on a variety of dimensions (Reid, Parsons, & Green, 2001). Recognizing these facts, in 2001 the Rehabilitation Services Administration revised the definition of what constitutes an employment outcome under the state vocational rehabilitation. The revised definition of employment outcome eliminated extended employment (i.e., sheltered workshops) and other types of employment in segregated settings as employment outcomes, thereby allowing only employment in integrated settings in the community as employment outcomes under this program.

Why, then, have so few organizations made the complete shift from facility-based to community-based services? One reason is fairly straightforward: There have been few incentives to do so. In a study of state vocational rehabilitation agencies in all 50 states and the District of Columbia (Novak, Rogan, Mank, & DiLeo, 2003), only 26 states reported fiscal incentives to provide supported employment over segregated day services. In addition, organizational change requires internal leadership, strong values favoring integration, long-term commitment, persistence, and creativity. Other barriers to organizational change include a basic fear and resistance to change and the unknown, negative, or apprehensive attitudes among stakeholders, conflicting policies and regulations (i.e., some impeding movement to integrated and individualized services), lack of expertise, transportation and attendant care issues, the need for trained staff, and the complexity of the change process (Fesko & Butterworth, 2001; Rogan, 2005).

Fortunately, a growing number of organizations have undertaken the complex process of organizational change, sometimes referred to as *conversion.* These organizations have demonstrated that the provision of services without walls (totally community-based services) is not only possible, but results in better outcomes for individuals and the organization itself (Brooks-Lane, Hutcheson, & Revell, 2005; Lawhead, 2005; Verstegan, 2005).

ORGANIZATIONAL CHANGE STUDIES

A number of publications have documented various aspects of the organizational change process experienced by service providers throughout the United States (Albin, Rhodes, & Mank, 1994; Beare, Severson, Lynch, & Schneider, 1992; Block, 1997; Fesko & Butterworth, 2001; Hagner & Murphy, 1989; Lawhead, 2005; Murphy & Rogan, 1995; Oldman Thomson, Calsaferri, Luke, & Bond, 2005; Parent, Hill, & Wehman, 1989; Rogan, Held, & Rinne, 2001; Walker, 2000). Although each organization is unique, common themes have emerged. Strategies for addressing the needs of various constituents (or customers), including people with disabilities, parents, agency staff, employers, co-workers, boards of directors, community living providers, and state and local funders, have been described (see Rogan, Held, & Rinne, 2001, for a complete discussion).

Common phases of change in any organization include:

- helping organizational members and stakeholders understand and accept the need for change
- developing a clear image or vision of the organization's possible future
- getting stakeholder buy-in for the change
- developing a strategic plan for change
- implementing the action plan
- monitoring outcomes and making adjustments accordingly

These phases establish the motivation, direction, and expectation for action across the organization. More specifically, studies of organizational change from facility-based to community-based services have included some or all of the following strategies.

Articulate a Clear Mission, Vision, and Values

The process of developing a new mission statement provides an ideal forum for discussing the vision and underlying values of the organization with key constituents. Doing so helps individuals better understand the need for change. A clearly articulated mission, vision, and values statement helps to avoid confusion and to clarify the new direction. The vision statement serves to articulate where the organization would like to be in the future. The values statement describes the beliefs that guide the organization's actions. The mission statement describes what the organization does. Organizational decisions need to be referenced against this mission statement and aligned with the vision and values of the organization.

Involve Key Stakeholders from the Start

Organizational change directly or indirectly impacts all of the people involved in, or associated with, the services of an organization. These stakeholders, including people with disabilities, parents, employment and residential agency personnel, funding agency personnel, case managers, employers, and board members, can work for or against the change. Organizations have learned the importance of pulling stakeholders into the discussions early in the change process. Each of these partner groups may require different approaches to assist them to understand and support the need for change. It is not likely that all stakeholders will support organizational change efforts. Some may be wed to the facility-based services and may actively resist any major changes.

Nevertheless, changeover efforts should proceed while efforts ensue to gain the support of resistant constituents.

Multiple strategies have been used to involve stakeholders in formal and informal ways. Many organizations form a change management team comprised of representatives from each main stakeholder group. This body steers the planning and change process, and is responsible for keeping their constituents informed and involved. Other organizations host forums and form work groups involving various interested parties. It is important to address directly the concerns among various stakeholders by providing a great deal of information and multiple discussion forums over time. Some organizations have learned that it is more effective to address individual family concerns on a one-to-one basis rather than meet with all parents in a large group meeting. It has also been effective to facilitate parent-to-parent meetings between parents who are strong advocates and reluctant or resistant parents.

Flatten the Organizational Structure

The organizational change process has significant implications for restructuring of the agency. As previously stated, organizations have typically added community services to their continuum without redesigning services or significantly impacting the organizational chart. Organizational change often involves restructuring to a flatter organizational structure. This involves eliminating some programs and positions in favor of streamlining services to focus heavily on integrated employment, moving more staff resources to direct service roles in the community, and rewriting job descriptions to reflect this employment emphasis. In other words, organizations that have converted have fewer layers in their hierarchy, and more staff positions involved in direct services in the community.

Build Strong Leadership from Within the Organization

Although organizational change has been driven primarily by internal executive directors and top level managers, organizations undertaking the changeover process benefit from leadership throughout the organization. A flattened organizational structure and redesigned job descriptions that move more decision-making power to front-line staff may facilitate this outcome. Ongoing staff development is critical to building a strong repertoire of skills and competence among staff members so they can make wise decisions and assume leadership roles within the organization.

Hire and Train Quality Staff

Organizations involved in the changeover to community services may have personnel who have worked at the facility for many years, and who may or may not be excited about the new direction. Some may leave voluntarily while others may be asked to leave. In some organizational change cases, there was up to 50% turnover in staff during the changeover process. When existing staff have been redeployed to provide community-based employment services, they have benefited from an extensive investment of information, training, and support on an ongoing basis. Organizations have capitalized on the opportunity to recruit and hire new staff with desired skills and positive attitudes about the capabilities of people with disabilities, integrated employment, and community membership. Rather than look for people who know about disability, many organizations have sought people who have business savvy; demonstrate strong initiative, problem solving, and social skills; and who are well connected to a particular community.

Empower Staff Through Teamwork

Since community services require agency personnel to work in dispersed community settings and largely in isolation from their colleagues, staff have appreciated opportunities to work in teams. Team structures have allowed staff to share roles and responsibilities, expertise, resources, and personal support. For example, a team of four employment specialists may share support responsibilities for 30–40 individuals who have differing needs for support. Within this team, the staff provide backup for each other as needed and support individuals throughout the day. Although there may be individual areas of expertise within the team, all team members may play a role in all aspects of the employment process (e.g., job development, job training, follow-along). Some organizations with flat structures have developed self-directed teams that manage most of their affairs and services. For example, self-directed teams

- Identify a team leader from within their team. This role can rotate among team members.

- Meet on a weekly basis to provide updates on the progress of the people they support, problem solve about issues that come up, review the weekly schedule and staff coverage needs, share information, and so forth.

- Hire new staff with desired expertise to complement and enhance existing team member strengths.

- Seek and provide feedback to each other on a regular basis regarding each staff member's professional development goals and performance.

Use Individualized, Holistic
Person-Centered Planning Approaches

Person-centered planning (PCP) has been a central tool for assisting individuals and their families to identify dreams, interests, and needs, and to develop action plans for achieving desired outcomes (Bradley, 1994; Forest & Lusthaus, 1990; Mount, 1992; Turnbull & Turnbull, 1992). PCP has also proven to be a powerful learning tool for agency personnel because it has helped staff get to know people and to view them from a strengths-based perspective. It is necessary to revisit action plans on a regular basis in order to maintain a sense of urgency to reach desired outcomes and to hold each team member accountable for various activities (Pearpoint, O'Brien, & Forest, 1993). Ultimately, consumer satisfaction is the key gauge to determine the effectiveness of the PCP process and outcomes.

Adopt a One-Person-at-a-Time Approach

Organizational change to community services requires a one-person-at-a-time approach. That is, an individualized approach is necessary to match people with jobs and other desired life outcomes (e.g., volunteer work, involvement in community organizations, use of community businesses) based on their unique interests and needs. Therefore, organizations need to avoid the temptation to move groups of people into enclaves and work crews as a quick-fix approach to community services. Enclaves and work crews reduce individualization, integration, and natural supports, and often skew the employer-employee relationship because the provider agency typically pays the workers. In addition, enclaves and work crews require a great deal of time and effort to disassemble when individualized jobs are preferred. Thus, organizations should attempt to do it right the first time by pursuing a one person–one job approach.

Start With Those Who Want Out

Typically, at least half of the individuals in sheltered workshops express an interest in getting a regular job in the community or in pursuing meaningful nonwork activities. These individuals should be the first to be supported to leave the facility. After this first wave of people, there will be others who decide they, too, are interested in getting a job. This pattern continues as wave after wave of individuals move out of the facility, providing demonstrations of success for reluctant individuals and family members. In the end, there may be a handful of individuals who are left in the facility, often due to parental resistance. Clearly, an entire facility is not needed to serve a handful of people, so closure of the facility should be imminent. Individualized plans are made by asking each person: How do you want to spend your day, with whom, and where?

Involve Individuals in Career Exploration Activities

Since many people have never worked in the community, they may not have a good understanding of job options or their own job interests. When asked what kind of job a person might like to do, it is natural for people to choose the type of work they have done in the workshop. In many cases, people are fearful of the unknown and have perceptions of the community as unsafe and non-supportive. In order to expand understanding of community employment opportunities, organizations should provide multiple job exploration experiences. Agencies can invite individuals to participate in job clubs, information interviews, job shadowing, job try-outs, volunteer work, temporary work, and other community activities. These experiences not only provide excellent assessment information, but they also allow individuals to get a feel for available opportunities, what they like or don't like, and help to de-mystify community employment.

Terminate Facility Admissions and Backfilling

At some point it becomes apparent to organizations in the midst of the organizational change process that it does not make sense to continue allowing people to be admitted to the facility, or to allow individuals to return to the facility if they lose their job (i.e., backfilling). The point at which this decision is made varies from agency to agency, and is one of the hardest to make. Some organizations allow individuals who lose their job to return to the workshop temporarily until another job is secured. This safety net may be viewed as important for individuals and their families in order to make it easier for them to try supported employment. Other agencies have not allowed people to return to the workshop, but instead developed an array of options for people who lose their job, as described in the next section.

Develop Safety Net Options for When People Lose Their Jobs

It is a given that some people will lose their job in the community for various reasons. Organizations need to plan for this occurrence from the start with individuals and family members. Options should be developed that include 1) participating in one's job hunt, 2) volunteering, 3) taking a relevant class (preferably in the community rather than at the facility), 4) participating in personally meaningful community activities, and/or 5) staying at home temporarily. Some organizations have secured job sites that are receptive to allowing someone to work there for a short time while another job is being sought. Returning to the facility should be considered a last-resort option, if at all.

Access External Consultants to Help Guide the Changeover Process

Organizations have found it helpful to invite external expertise to assist in planning and implementation efforts because organizational change is a challenging process. Sometimes a neutral outsider can say things that internal leaders cannot, or can reinforce messages that have already been given. Sometimes people within the organization are so close to the issues that they cannot see problems, solutions, or progress. During the changeover process there are plateau periods when organizations feel stuck. A fresh set of eyes and perspectives can help organizations gauge their progress and identify next steps for moving forward. Another approach for accessing external expertise is to send staff to visit other organizations that have already undertaken the changeover process. By doing this, staff can actually see the outcomes of change efforts and can learn from multiple people who have walked the walk.

Change the Agency's Image Through Marketing

Organizations that had been known for providing sheltered services in their communities need to market themselves differently to the business community. Instead of being viewed as the place where "those" people go, and where employers send their work, organizations want to be seen as a viable source of workers to meet employer's needs. Marketing materials often need to be redesigned to better reflect a business and employment orientation, rather than a human services disability perspective. Agencies with names such as "Sunnyville Program for the Retarded" or "Handicapable Hands" must also change their names to better represent their new focus.

Build Business Partnerships

Organizational change typically requires different relationships with the business community. At some point, subcontract work will no longer be brought into the facility, so business relationships need to be reoriented to a hiring-and-support focus. Agencies should consider forming a business advisory council comprised of a small group of area employers to assist in designing and disseminating marketing materials to the business community. Ideally, members of this group should be employers who have hired individuals with disabilities and are positive about this experience. They can be asked to speak with other employers to promote supported employment.

Divest of Buildings and Equipment

As significant numbers of people move out of the facility into community employment, it makes sense for organizations to divest of their buildings and equipment. Multiple options can be pursued, depending on whether the organization owned, rented, or leased the building(s), vehicles, and equipment. Unloading these "sunk costs" can provide a source of income for the organization (Hannan & Freeman, 1984).

Pursue Flexible Funding and Alternative Sources of Funds

In many cases, funding has been a barrier to organizational change. Funding structures have supported facility-based services based on a group orientation to service delivery. Organizations have found it necessary to renegotiate funding structures to allow for individualized services and supports. For example, an agency may prefer block funding (receiving funding in one lump sum) so that funds can be distributed as needed, or hourly rate funding so that true costs are covered. In addition, organizations have sought to diversify their funding sources so they are not as dependent on state funding. For example, agencies may opt to provide services for Welfare to Work recipients in order to tap that funding source. State developmental disability (DD) councils and state agencies (e.g., vocational rehabilitation, DD) have offered bridge funding to organizations to cover the period of time when both sheltered and community-based programs are operating. In rare cases, state agencies and a DD council have pooled resources to support a state organizational change effort. Finally, some organizations have acquired grants from national, state, and private funding sources to support their efforts.

Showcase and Celebrate Success

It is important for agencies to showcase their successes internally as well as in the larger community because organizational change is relatively new, challenging, and controversial for many organizations. For example, newsletter and newspaper articles that feature positive stories help to inform constituents and impact attitudes and perceptions. Staff can earn kudos and perks for accomplishing desired outcomes. The agency can host get-togethers to thank employers or celebrate supported employee accomplishments. Too often, agencies are so busy providing services that they neglect these important celebrations. They have proven to be essential to the health and well-being of organizations in order to develop a positive climate and maintain morale over time.

OUTCOMES OF ORGANIZATIONAL CHANGE

In one of the few investigations that evaluated the outcomes of organizational change, Murphy et al. (2002) conducted a qualitative study of the situations and perspectives of people with disabilities eight years after facility conversion. The 16 study participants were blind or visually impaired and had multiple disability classifications, including mental retardation, cerebral palsy, psychiatric disabilities, and deafness. There appeared to be no relationship between disability labels and outcomes. Fifteen of the 16 individuals secured at least one competitive job after leaving the facility, with an average of 2.5 jobs each and a range of 1–5 jobs. All individuals earned more than minimum wage and all worked less than full time. At the time of the interviews, five people were not working and some had waited long periods for another chance to work. Thirteen of the 16 people were positive about the closure of the facility. The others experienced service delays and inadequacies that caused them stress and anxiety. That is, funding decisions favored new applicants and initial placements, rather than job replacements. In contrast, people entering sheltered facilities faced no delays. This situation reflected the conflicting funding messages and regulations that continue to favor sheltered services.

The strategies described above are common but not universal in the organizational change process. Each organization is unique and must determine a pathway that makes sense in their circumstances. The case study described below provides an in-depth examination of the changeover efforts of one organization. This description highlights key beliefs, values, practices, barriers, and outcomes in the journey toward meaningful lives for those receiving services.

JAY NOLAN COMMUNITY SERVICES

The following in-depth example of one agency's organizational change journey over the last decade illustrates the complexity of the process and the many challenges and rewards inherent in such a transformational change. Jay Nolan Community Services (JNCS) was founded in 1975 by a group of families who were associated with the Autism Society of Los Angeles (ASLA). In the early 1970s, families who had children with autism had only two viable options: to keep their child at home with very little support, or institutionalize their child. No other real options existed. JNCS was formed because other organizations in the Los Angeles area failed to serve people with autism primarily because of their behavioral challenges. The main goal of JNCS was to serve those people who were not accepted in any other community program, and to provide state of the art services for people with autism. From the beginning, JNCS adopted a zero rejection policy, meaning that people's behavior could not get them rejected from services, and parents and families were involved in all facets of decision making.

In 1975, JNCS opened a Saturday program. The goal of this program was to allow people with autism to do something on a Saturday away from their families, providing a break to the family, and hopefully to allow growth and fun for the individual. This was provided in a central site for six hours each weekend. It was a fairly traditional program in terms of the activities that were provided.

In 1976, JNCS opened its first group home followed shortly by a second group home. JNCS always had a commitment to bringing people out of the state hospital as well as serving people from the community. The group homes demonstrated this commitment by ensuring that an equal percentage of people in the group homes were community people and others were from the state hospital. The group homes lead to the beginning of a workshop in a garage of one of the group homes, providing woodworking experiences to the people in that group home. Over the years the number of group homes and day programs grew.

By 1988, Jay Nolan had opened 10 more group homes and had a total of three traditional day programs, which were actually behavior management programs. These day programs were facility-based and focused on activities typical of such programs across the country. Work was never a real priority. The group homes served about 65 people and the day programs served approximately 120 people.

In 1989, JNCS moved from providing site-based day programs to beginning to provide three community-based behavioral day programs. These were mainly enclaves in the community involving flyer delivery, ground maintenance, and gardening. This was an attempt to move people out of the site-based programs into the community for all or part of each day. Also in 1989, JNCS began to provide supported employment with funding from the Department of Rehabilitation for a very small number of people who had less challenging needs.

By 1990, JNCS moved from providing traditional site-based day programs to providing, for lack of another name, van therapy programs in the community. People started each day at the day program site, but were in the community for the majority of the day. Most people were placed in a small group (1:2 or 1:3 ratio) and spent their days driving around or visiting places such as parks, malls, zoos, or beaches. While some people had something that looked like part-time employment, the vast majority of people were unemployed, and employment was not viewed as a real option for many others.

In 1992, a crisis struck JNCS that involved fiscal problems, a lack of trust between the board of directors, the management/administration, and the ASLA board. This led to the removal of the executive director. The executive director was loved by many people and with his departure came tension, distrust, and fear. An independent evaluation was conducted in July 1992 by a group of external local and national experts. The evaluation report entitled "A Moment in Time: An Agency in Crisis" described that while everyone cared about the people being served, their lives were not very good.

As a result, the board of directors initiated a search for a new executive director. An individual who was part of the evaluation team, Jeff Strully, was asked to apply and ultimately was hired in 1993. After the hiring of the new executive director, JNCS started to change the way of doing business. The organization wanted to move toward supporting people to lead more inclusive, richer, fuller, and personalized lives.

Change Begins at JNCS

Change began initially with the group homes. Between 1993 and 1995, JNCS closed 13 group homes. People were supported to move to their own places one person at a time with a "whatever it takes" attitude. This occurred by empowering people with disabilities, their families, support personnel, and allies. It also involved person-centered planning and using circles of support to guide the efforts. At the same time, there was a move to begin closing the site-based day programs and to move away from grouping people and utilizing vans.

This change began by picking people up and dropping them off in generic locations (e.g., at their home, in the park, at a restaurant). People who knew the individual and who were in support roles (e.g., family members, staff, friends) were brought together as a circle of support for each person. They collaborated with the individual to design daily schedules. Each individual and their circle of support members (though in reality many people didn't have and still don't have a complete circle) were asked to design their own daily schedule. How would they like to spend their day? What would they like to do and with whom? Each person's schedule had the following components:

A meeting place in the community that made sense for each individual where agency support started and ended each day. This is normally one's home, however, from time to time this may have been a restaurant or another community location.

Back-up plans were developed for all of the "what if" situations that might arise. Issues such as inclement weather, or if staff were to become ill or not show up, were addressed to be sure there were contingency plans in place.

Cross-training plans were essential so that more than one staff member knew each person, their schedule, and the respective community sites that they frequented. Thus, a primary and secondary staff person was identified for each person.

Crisis support plans were developed for instances when people with behavior challenges needed significant support. Since staff worked and supported people on their own in the community, it was critical that they had the necessary skills and plans to respond to such situations.

Vocational profiles were developed with and for all individuals, whether they were working or not, to document work history, interests, support needs, possible job matches, and so forth. These were used by staff to guide job development and other related activities.

Finally, during this transitional time, the family support component of the organization was also involved in the redesign of services from group and congregate approaches to more personalized and individualized supports. This included the ending of several programs and the beginning of several new program components, which supported children and young adults with autism to join local associations (church, civic clubs, social clubs, YMCA).

Changing Old Ways of Thinking and Doing

The management team developed a vision for the organization using the Planning Alternative Tomorrows with Hope (PATH) planning tool (Pearpoint, O'Brien, & Forest, 1993). In the first few years, JNCS invested in many outside consultants to help change the mindset of parents, staff, and others. This mass education on the value of inclusion was conducted throughout the organization.

One of the primary changes was an attempt to help people with disabilities get away from the world of disability, which was controlled by human services professionals aimed at segregation, labels, and boxed treatment. Center-based services were predicated on the following: lack of choices, exclusion, chaos, artificial structure, limitations, systems-centered services, power over relationships, quality assurance being defined by rules and regulations, decisions made by the organization, assumed incompetence, and a need to "treat" people. The biggest challenge was to change the mindset of staff and families. There was resistance, fear, and anger about these changes.

Over time, staff roles changed in order to better support people. For example, the staff were encouraged to be more responsible and autonomous, listen to people rather than control them, promote community connections, and to support only those with whom they had a relationship and common interests. This shift to a person-centered approach was a real challenge for most staff. Many people left the organization and others paid lip service to the change. Some staff who were involved in this process of making a shift went through stages of change themselves. That is, staff may have resisted changes initially, but over time an "aha!" moment of understanding and a commitment to change occurred.

This shift in mindset reflected a shift in values. The values that were reinforced included letting go of control; avoiding labels; using one's own life as a yardstick; giving and getting (i.e., reciprocation) genuine relationships; speaking with, not for, people; power with rather than power over people; and learning to listen, accept, respect, and love.

The shifting of the culture to person-centered day supports meant more choices and empowerment for people and their families, increased inclusion and consistency in people's day and routines, real life experiences in the community, services designed around the person, circles of support, increased use of generic community resources, assumed competence, and more holistic approaches to people's lives.

Values that Guide JNCS

JNCS has a deep commitment to a set of values and beliefs that guide all decisions and services. These include:

1. All people have capacity and gifts.

2. People need a sense of belonging to their community.

3. People can contribute to the community.

4. Relationships and trust are equally fundamental for inclusion to happen.

5. All people can live in their own homes with the right supports.

6. All people should be treated with dignity and respect.

7. Self-advocacy and empowerment should be promoted.

8. The health and safety of people is paramount.

9. All people have the right to be free from pain, coercion, and cruelty.

10. All people have the right to be heard and their ideas acknowledged.

It is easy for an organization to say what they believe. The hard part is living these values on a daily basis. An organization and individual support circles need to be challenged when they don't live up to these values. There are no simple solutions to complex human problems. However, organizations need to be guided by their values and beliefs. JNCS has tried over its entire history to live up to its values and to rethink its value system as changes in the world took place.

Tools for Change

Creating change in an organization requires a tool box. The more tools in the box, the more likely you are going to be successful. The following tools have helped create change at JCNS.

1. *Circles of support*—This involves the gathering of a group of people who are committed to the individual, are willing to help figure out what is needed, and are willing to struggle with the difficult and troubling questions. While the organization continues to struggle with this, circles of support are key to figuring out who people are and what they want to do with their lives.

2. *Use of MAPS/PATH planning tools*—While there are many planning tools (e.g., Essential Lifestyle Planning, PCP), JCNS has utilized Making Action Plans (MAPs) and PATH to learn more about the individual—who they are, what they want, what works, and so forth. These planning tools have assisted in the journey to better understand those whom the agency supports. These planning tools are grounded in the assumption that a desirable future is possible, each individual has a voice and gifts and is central to the process, and that it can't be achieved alone or in a vacuum.

3. *Intentionality*—Valued lives in the community will not just happen because we want it to happen. They happen because we have worked on it. People will more likely have the type of life they want if the people close to them purposefully work to make it happen and maintain a sense of urgency in the process.

4. *Facilitation*—Along with intentionality, facilitation is required to assist and support each person in moving forward with his or her dreams. The role of a support person is not just to do, but to facilitate such things as natural supports and greater independence.

5. *Community building*—Being in the community is not the same as being part of the community. Many people with disabilities are physically present in the community, but they are not connected. JNCS believes that people need to be connected to a network of neighbors, friends, co-workers, and other community members.

Linda's Story

Linda is a 38-year-old woman described as having self-injurious and obsessive/ compulsive behaviors, constant agitation, inappropriate social behavior—frequently assaultive and causing property destruction —severe cognitive disabilities, autism, and poor communication and self-help skills. At this time, Linda was in crisis at her group home and in her workshop day program. She was biting herself and others about eight times a week. These bites generally required medical treatment. She put her head through a wall and required stitches. She tore her closet door off and broke her arm in two places. She smashed a window at her group home. She spent her entire day in the workshop. Staff believed she was too out of control to be in the community. Her circle of support decided to develop a plan to begin to integrate her into the community because she was so isolated.

When the circle came together to plan with Linda about her life, the first question was "Who is Linda?" She was described as loving, fun, neat, charming, smart, flirtatious, stubborn, and adventurous. She was viewed as a "daddy's girl" and "tough chick" who loves rock and roll, tests limits, communicates clearly without words, knows what she wants, and loves the beach and horses. Initially, Linda required two staff to be with her in the community. After a year, Linda was supported on a 1:1 ratio and was fully integrated in the community, including moving into her own home.

Between 1993 and 1995, Linda's circle developed numerous jobs for her. She worked at a Pizza Hut. This didn't last long, as Linda couldn't understand why she had to give the pizza away. She tried working at Foster Freeze, but she didn't like wearing the hat. A courier delivery service was then developed for her with a nonprofit employer. She got laid off. Today, Linda works at Sports Chalet 30 hours a week where she does mainly stocking, pricing, and carrying out bags for customers. She has medical benefits through her employer and difficult behaviors are rarely seen. Linda's day support staff have been with her for over 4 years.

Outcomes of JNCS Personalized Day Supports

People's lives have changed significantly as the attitudes, values, and practices of JNCS staff have changed. People now live with significantly less violence in their lives as a result of living in their own home. Expenditures on repairs and maintenance have decreased since group homes were closed. People are more in control over who supports them. Some people are spending their days with only one other person, who has the same interests and goals. People initiate more and have more choices and influence in their lives, and are having the opportunity to experience sharing ordinary community places. People have shown unexpected resilience and adaptability, and are contributing to their communities.

Defining Personalized Day Support   What is personalized day support? Simply put, it is about each person, not a group of people. It is about flexible supports in order to meet people's needs and desires. It is about getting support to do what you need and want to do during the day. It is about helping people develop valued social roles, autonomy and independence to the greatest extent possible. It is about inclusion, not exclusion, in the community and shifting control from staff to the consumer. It is about having fun and about getting a life!

The following are some of the guidelines JNCS used to help people have meaningful days

1. *Start with the values.* Everything must start with the values and beliefs as shared previously. These values and beliefs must guide your actions and if compromises are made, they are made knowing that you are making a compromise. There is a difference between compromising and selling out.

2. *Develop a vision that recognizes socially valued roles.* Each of the people receiving support needs to have opportunities for socially valued roles: worker, friend, lover, learner, student, volunteer, explorer, and so forth.

3. *Identify who the person is and what they need, desire, and want.* The more you know who this person is, the better support can be provided.

4. *Implement the vision.* Simply put, ready, aim, fire! Okay, maybe that gets you in trouble, but you have to take a leap from time to time and just do it. If it fails, then get up and do it again another way. There are no simple solutions or easy ways to make this happen other than trying, learning, and doing.

5. *Track and identify outcomes to maintain direction.* This is not always easy for organizations. Organizations have maintained a "we know best" attitude and have a long history of telling people to trust them. Tracking individual outcomes may include work hours, wages, benefits, degree of integration, nature of natural supports, social relationships, and other quality of life issues. Ultimately, data need to tell us how we are doing and whether the people hiring us (people with disabilities and the funders) are getting their money's worth.

6. *Think in terms of competency building and image enhancement.* The more valued roles that people have, the more valued they are viewed.

7. *The people who support the people are important.* Staff need to know what they are doing and why, and they need to be compensated and rewarded so that they will be there over time.

Challenges of the Journey

While great strides have been made over the years at JNCS, there is still much to be done. Maybe the journey is really never over, but continues to evolve over time. These are some of the greatest challenges at JNCS in the past decade:

1. **Funding**—If you don't receive enough resources, it is difficult to hire, retain, and reward good employees. It is challenging for organizations if there are more expectations from funders without additional revenue to cover training, supervision, back-up support, crisis intervention, and so on.

2. **Individuals served by other organizations**—Some consumers supported by JNCS during the day are still living in group homes operated by other organizations. This leads to many challenging issues about differing values, control, empowerment, schedules, supports, and risks.

3. **Employment discrimination**—Although the Americans with Disabilities Act (1990), Section 504 of the Rehabilitation Act of 1973 (PL 93-112), and many other legal provisions exist to protect workers with disabilities, discrimination still exists. It may be difficult to prove that you are being discriminated against. Individuals face continued employment discrimination every day in the real world.

4. **When 1:1 support is not possible**—Matching consumers together in 1:2 or 1:3 ratios can be very difficult. What is the best way to do it? Who should be paired? When? Under what circumstances? What are the unintended consequences of such decisions? Are there alternatives, assuming natural supports have been tapped?

5. **Tensions with state funding agencies**—Organizations typically rely on state funding from MR/DD, vocational rehabilitation (VR), or mental health agencies. Although VR should be the agency that people who are working are connected with, at least initially, many VR offices reject the vast majority of people with high support needs. This is because VR expects people to demonstrate a reduction in support needs over time. Some may not meet this expectation. If individuals always need support, VR may expect them to be in enclaves, work crews and mobile crews, rather than individualized employment. This causes tension between the provider and VR.

6. **Jobs with benefits**—Developing jobs that have benefits such as medical, vacation, and 401(k), can be difficult. For the most part, JNCS is still securing employment that is entry level. This has caused JNCS to reflect on its actions, and to challenge individual circles of support to raise the bar and seek better jobs.

7. **Staffing**—Because JNCS is so personalized in their supports, back-up is especially difficult if someone is off because of illness or vacation. Depending upon the individual, this could cause a disruption in their schedule. It can also change the quality of support. Some people have extensive support back-up and others have few people involved.

8. **Shifting parent's mindset toward fading**—Put another way, families have fought for and come to expect 1:1 support. Some believe their son or daughter requires higher levels of support than might actually be needed. However, for a variety of reasons, parents may view a reduction of support as bad. However, as stated above, unless fading occurs, VR funding for supported employment is very difficult to secure, if not impossible. In addition, funding for ongoing supports may never be sufficient for 1:1 ratios.

9. **Assisting people to have meaningful and ordinary lives**—This is easier said than done. Barriers, including history, community attitudes, staff

competency, and fear interfere with full inclusion of people with significant disabilities in our communities. Thinking outside the box does not come easily for many people.

JNCS has accomplished much over the past nine years. However, there is much more work to be done before the organization will be satisfied. People with disabilities are not working in careers and don't have as much money as they need. They don't have lots of friends and other relationships. People don't own their own homes, and have to rely on paid providers to support them. However, the journey will continue.

We may never get to the place we really want to be. But what is the alternative—not to do it because of the challenges? NO. Can we wait for the answers and then things will be perfect? NO. So, we try. We fail. We make mistakes. We are trying to change the day-to-day life experiences of very devalued and wounded people in our society. That is not going to happen overnight, nor is it going to be simple. However, it is worth working on because the people we care about are worth it.

CONCLUSION

This chapter highlighted the status of organizational change nationally, and described multiple barriers and change strategies. The example of JNCS is exciting because, as a large agency serving people with significant challenges, it has undertaken a major organizational shift. In the United States, traditional providers serve the vast majority of people with developmental disabilities. Unless these providers change, the lives of the people being served will not change. Unless parents see a new future for their son or daughter, self-determination will not happen for many people. Unless there are people willing to stand with people who challenge us, those with high support needs will remain segregated, dependent, undervalued, limited in their potential, and denied full citizenship.

People's lives and life circumstances are complex and very challenging, as is organizational change. Yet, great satisfaction comes from working with individuals toward regular lives and true community membership. We know the barriers and have learned many valuable strategies. Others have successfully accomplished organizational change and demonstrated that we do not need facilities that congregate and segregate people. Our field knows better. All we need now is committed leadership for systems change and a stronger effort to invite the involvement of our generic communities in this endeavor.

REFERENCES

Albin, J., Rhodes, L., & Mank, D. (1994). Realigning organizational culture, resources, and community roles: Changeover to community employment. *Journal of the Association for Persons with Severe Handicaps, 19*, 105–115.

Americans with Disabilities Act of 1990, PL 101-336, 42 U.S.C. §§ 12101 *et seq.*

Beare, P.L., Severson, S.J., Lynch, E.C., & Schneider, D. (1992). Small agency conversion to community-based employment: Overcoming the barriers. *Journal for Persons with Severe Handicaps, 17,* 170–178.

Block, S.R. (1997). Closing the sheltered workshop: Toward competitive employment opportunities for persons with developmental disabilities. *Journal of Vocational Rehabilitation, 9*(3), 267–275.

Braddock, D., Rizzolo, M., & Hemp, R. (2004). Most employment services growth in developmental disabilities during 1988–2002 was in segregated settings. *Mental Retardation, 42*(4), 317–320.

Bradley, V. (1994). Evolution of a new service paradigm. In V. Bradley, J. Ashbaugh, and B. Blaney (Eds.), *Creating individual supports for people with developmental disabilities* (pp. 11–32). Baltimore: Paul H. Brookes Publishing Co.

Brooks-Lane, N., Hutcheson, S., & Revell, G. (2005). Supporting consumer directed employment outcomes. *Journal of Vocational Rehabilitation, 23*(2), 123–134.

Butterworth, J., Metzel, D., Boeltzig, H., Gilmore, D., & Sulweski, J. (2005, May/June). Employment outcomes: Room for change. *TASH Connections, 31*(5/6).

Fesko, S., & Butterworth, J. (Eds.) (2001). *Conversion to integrated employment: Case studies of organizational change.* Boston: Institute for Community Inclusion, Children's Hospital, University of Massachusetts, Boston.

Forest, M., & Lusthaus, E. (1990). Everyone belongs with MAPS action planning system. *Teaching Exceptional Children, 22,* 32–35.

Gilmore, D., & Butterworth, J. (1996). *Work status trends for people with mental retardation.* Boston: Institute for Community Inclusion.

Hagner, D., & Murphy, S. (1989). Closing the shop on sheltered work: Case studies of organizational change. *Journal of Rehabilitation, 55*(3), 68–74.

Hannan, M., & Freeman, J. (1984). Structural inertia and organizational change. *American Sociological Review, 49*(2), 149–164.

Hernandez, B., Keys, C., & Balcazar, F. (2002). Employer attitudes toward workers with disabilities and their Americans with Disabilities Act employment rights: A literature review. *Journal of Rehabilitation, 66,* 4–16.

Kiernan, W., & Schalock, W. (Eds.) (1997). *Integrated employment: Current status and future directions.* Washington, DC: American Association on Mental Retardation.

Lawhead, B. (2005). Opportunities for too few? Oversight of federal employment programs for people with disabilities. *The Advance, 16*(3). Richmond, VA: APSE, The Network on Employment.

Mank, D. (1994). The underachievement of supported employment: A call for reinvestment. *Journal of Disability Policy Studies, 5*(2), 1–24.

Mank, D., Cioffi, A., & Yovanoff, P. (2003). Supported employment outcomes across a decade: Is there evidence of improvement in the quality of implementation? *Mental Retardation, 41*(3), 188–197.

McCaughrin, W., Ellis, W., Rusch, F., & Heal, L. (1993). Cost-effectiveness of supported employment. *Mental Retardation, 31*(1), 41–48.

Migliore, A., Mank, D., Grossi, T., & Rogan, P. (in press). Integrated employment or sheltered workshops: Preferences of adults with intellectual disabilities, their families, and staff. *Journal of Vocational Rehabilitation, 26*(1).

Mount, B. (1992). *Person-centered planning: Finding directions for change using personal futures planning.* New York: Graphics Futures, Inc.

Murphy, S., & Rogan, P. (1995). *Closing the shop: Conversion from sheltered to integrated work.* Baltimore: Paul H. Brookes Publishing Co.

Murphy, S., Rogan, P., Hanley, M., Kincaid, C., & Royce-Davis, J. (2002). People's situations and perspectives 8 years after workshop conversion. *Mental Retardation, 40*(1), 30–40.

Novak, J., Rogan, P., Mank, D., & DiLeo, D. (2003). Supported employment and systems change: Findings from a national survey of state vocational rehabilitation agencies. *Journal of Vocational Rehabilitation, 19*(3), 157–166.

Oldman, J., Thomson, L., Calsaferri, K., Luke, A., & Bond, G. (2005). A case report of the conversion of sheltered employment to evidence-based supported employment in Canada. *Psychiatric Services, 56*(11), 1436–1440.

Parent, W., Hill, M., & Wehman, P. (1989). From sheltered to supported employment outcomes: Challenges for rehabilitation facilities. *Journal of Rehabilitation, 55*(4).

Pearpoint, J., O'Brien, J., & Forest, M. (1993). *Planning alternative tomorrows with hope: A workbook for planning better futures.* Toronto: Center for Integrated Education and Communities.

Rehabilitation Act of 1973, PL 93-112, 29 U.S.C. §§ 701 *et seq.*

Reid, D.H., Parsons, M.B., & Green, C.W. (2001). Evaluating the functional utility of congregate day treatment activities for adults with severe disabilities. *American Journal on Mental Retardation, 106,* 460–469.

Rogan, P. (2005). Moving from segregation to integration: Organizational change strategies and outcomes. In P. Wehman, V. Brooke, K. Inge, & G. Revell (Eds.), *Inclusive employment: Persons with disabilities going to work.* Baltimore: Paul H. Brookes Publishing Co.

Rogan, P., Grossi, T., Mank, D., Haynes, D., Thomas, F., & Majd, C. (2001). *Changes in wage, hour, benefit, and integration outcomes of former sheltered workshop participants who are in supported employment.* Report for the President's Task Force on the Employment of Adults with Disabilities. Indiana University: Institute on Disability and Community.

Rogan, P., Held, M., & Rinne, S. (2001). Organizational change from sheltered to integrated employment for adults with disabilities. In P. Wehman (Ed.), *Supported employment in business: Expanding the capacity of workers with disabilities.* St. Augustine, FL: Training Resource Network, Inc.

Rusch, F., & Braddock, D. (2004). Adult day programs versus supported employment (1988–2002): Spending and service practices of mental retardation and developmental disabilities state agencies. *Research and Practice for Persons with Severe Disabilities, 29,* 237–242.

Taylor, S.J. (1988). Caught in the continuum: A critical analysis of the principle of the least restrictive environment. *The Journal of the Association of Persons with Severe Handicaps, 13*(1), 41–53.

Thompson, T.L., Powers, G., & Houchard, B. (1992). The wage effects of supported employment. *The Journal of the Association of Persons with Severe Handicaps, 17*(2), 85–94.

Turnbull, A., & Turnbull, R. (1992, Fall/Winter). Group action planning. *Families and Disability Newsletter,* 1–13.

Verstegan, D. (2005, Fall). Preparing for and implementing organizational change: Building more community employment opportunities. *Around the Region RSA Region V CRP-RCEP Newsletter, 10,* 1–5.

Walker, P. (2000). *Acting on a vision: Agency conversion at KFI, Millinocket, Maine.* Syracuse, NY: Center on Human Policy.

Wehman, P., & Bricout, J. (1999). Supported employment: Critical issues and new directions. *The impact of supported employment for people with significant disabilities: Preliminary findings from the National Supported Employment Consortium.* Richmond, VA: Virginia Commonwealth University RRTC on Workplace Supports.

Wehman, P., Revell, G. & Kregel, J. (1998). Supported employment: A decade of rapid growth and impact. *American Rehabilitation, 24*(1), 31–43.

CHAPTER NINE

Toward Meaningful Lives

A Convergence of Events, Problems, and Possibilities

DAVID M. MANK AND PATRICIA ROGAN

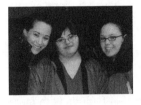 Meaningful lives: living, working, learning, and socializing where you want, when you want, and with whom you want. Having choices, speaking for yourself, and always reserving the right to change your mind. These are concepts increasingly familiar to people with disabilities, their families and friends, and those who work to support them. These are simple concepts as the harbingers of everyday living for every citizen. They are profound concepts, as it takes such purposeful effort to gain some semblance of their presence in the lives of people with significant disabilities.

This book has been about what is possible, and indeed, about what is taking place across the United States and around the world for people with significant disabilities. The early years of this millennium are marked by optimism about what is possible in everyday lives and continued concern about the halting pace of making meaningful lives a reality for all people with disabilities.

The context for the future appears to frame an unusual mix, even a convergence, of events, problems, and opportunities as the mission of support for people with disabilities becomes even clearer. Clarity from self-advocates and in government policy points increasingly to the now familiar components of meaningful lives: real work, a typical living situation, true friends, a social life, and access to the wealth of opportunities our communities provide for all their citizens. Nonetheless, serious problems exist that seemingly defy the clarity of direction of now well-established policy. At the same time, the quality and clarity of ideas and innovations provide continued hope for improvement. This final chapter explores this convergence of events, problems, and possibilities, and concludes with recommendations for necessary and bold changes that must occur to change outdated policies and practices.

CHALLENGES RELATED TO MEANINGFUL DAYTIMES

As reported in Chapter 3, national employment outcomes for adults with disabilities continue to be poor. Readers will recall the following synopsis of current national employment data and may share the following sentiments regarding this status.

- How can it be that more than 80% of people with disabilities are unemployed or underemployed in our country, and this statistic has not changed significantly in over a decade (Taylor, 2000)?

- Why do approximately 75% of vocational and day program participants receive services in sheltered employment, day activity, or day habilitation programs (Braddock, Hemp, & Rizzolo, 2005; Butterworth, Fesko, & Ma, 2000; Rizzolo, Hemp, Braddock, & Pomeranz-Essley, 2004)?

- Why is the trend in supported employment slowing while the rate of placements in segregated facilities is growing?

- Why is there still continued substantial state level investment in facility-based options (Dreilinger, Gilmore, & Butterworth, 2001; Migliore, Mank, Grossi, & Rogan, in press; Wehman, Revell, & Brooke, 2003)?

- Why are people with developmental disabilities overrepresented in segregated options and underrepresented in integrated options (Metzel, Butterworth, & Gilmore, 2004)?

- Why hasn't supported employment, which was designed for people with the most significant disabilities, served more than 7% of adults with more severe disabilities (Mank, Cioffi, & Yovanoff, 1998)?

- Why are there such wide variations in supported employment expenditures and outcomes from state to state (Braddock et al., 2004)?

- Why has supported employment underdelivered on its promise, with people working fewer than 25 hours per week on average (Murphy, Rogan, Handley, Kincaid, & Royce-Davis, 2002)?

- Why is there continued underfunding of initial (vocational rehabilitation [VR]) and long-term supports in order to ensure long-term employment success (Murphy et al., 2002)?

Changes in Policy

In the past, policies, legislation, court cases, and administration initiatives have often been in conflict (internally and with each other), about the direction of supports and services for people with significant disabilities (Taylor, 1988; Wehman et al., 2003). Policies supporting segregation have coexisted, sometimes without much friction, with policies declaring that people with disabilities really do have the same rights and responsibilities as everyone else (e.g., Mank, 1994). Now, there is increasing alignment of policy, law and funding, and legal action.

As stated in Chapter 1, the Americans with Disabilities Act (ADA) of 1990 (PL 101-336) continues to survive in its core message, even as lawsuits question some aspects. The ADA, along with the Individuals with Disabilities Education Improvement Act of 2004 (PL 108-446) and the Rehabilitation Act of 1973 (PL 93-112), creates a clear message of full participation of every citizen with disabilities. These and other legislation have continued to morph over time, yet in the same direction of full participation in fully integrated settings. In addition, executive branch initiatives and judicial action are in support of more personalized choices and outcomes (e.g., Wehman et al., 2005).

The New Freedom Initiative, developed by the Bush administration, seeks to provide incentives to states and communities to reduce segregation and to insure that money follows people from setting to setting (U.S. Department of Health & Human Services, 2001). This initiative is powerful as it supports a clear change in the relationship between people with disabilities and those who provide supports or services. That is, people with disabilities become decision makers about how resources are spent, rather than simply sent to a program funded directly by government.

The Olmstead decision (*Olmstead v. L.C. and E.W., 1999*) and the events it continues to cause in states align the direction of individual choices about the use of resources. It started as a single legal case about whether people in institutions had a choice to leave and whether money could follow the person. Not too many years ago such a notion was considered fairly radical. Now, the notion of money following people has the support of the Supreme Court, a court considered to be increasingly conservative in its views. Furthermore, now every state is expected to have a plan to reintegrate people with disabilities into communities. In addition, the Olmstead decision is now cited as a foundation for a lawsuit in Wisconsin focused on integrated employment and rejecting segregated employment (Pledl, 2005).

Lawsuits about waiting lists for supports and services have surfaced in a number of states. These lawsuits challenge the legality of the existence of waiting lists for services and most of these lawsuits are being settled out of court. These lawsuits are about access and, conceiveably, greater acceptance of people with disabilities as full citizens entitled to meaningful lives and to the supports that make possible meaningful lives and full participation.

The Medicaid Waiver program in Centers for Medicare & Medicaid Services (CMS) is becoming occasionally friendly to more fully support community participation *and* employment outcomes. Until recent years, little CMS money supported integrated day activity, as it was historically assigned to segregated settings. Over time, it became possible for states to write their waivers in a way that supported more community activity. Now, it is allowable and possible to support employment in real jobs in everyday businesses with Medicaid funding. Possibilities are emerging that CMS may request and support employment outcomes rather than simply allow employment supports as funded activities. In addition, the fact that CMS money "follows the person" means that it aligns with the calls from self-advocates and emerging government policy for control of resources.

Employment initiatives have emerged from perhaps unexpected places in government. Historically, initiatives for employment of people with disabilities have been largely the work of the Rehabilitation Services Administration (RSA), but this is no longer the case. The Clinton administration created The President's Committee on the Employment of People with Disabilities (Rogan, Grossi, Mark, Haynes, & Thomas, 2001), which clearly articulated the superiority of integration, wage, and benefit outcomes of supported employment compared to sheltered employment. The second Bush administration's New Freedom Initiative (U.S. Department of Health & Human Services, 2001) supports integrated employment. In the 1990s, the Department of Labor created the Office of Disability Employment Policy, which promotes real work in real businesses. Demonstration projects have emerged, creating renewed focus on decent employment and quality of life choices and outcomes. The Social Security Administration now emphasizes employment outcomes as it realizes that employment is the path to reduced Social Security Trust Fund expenditures. The Ticket to Work and Workforce Incentives Improvement Act of 1999 (PL 106-170) and the Medicaid Buy-In option, are creating incentives for providers to assist people with disabilities to secure and keep nearly full time employment. These efforts, along with the historical RSA focus on employment, and in addition to emerging CMS funding for employment, combine to create a stronger and clearer emphasis on integrated employment.

Reauthorizations of the Individuals with Disability Education Act and the Rehabilitation Act have focused, at least in some ways, on integrated employment, including transition from school to work. Over time, additional reauthorizations should provide other opportunities to ensure that legislation increasingly assures meaningful daytimes.

Perhaps for the first time, decisions by all three branches of government began to emerge that align in the direction of integrated daytime opportunities and employment. This increasing alignment of message and focus might make it possible to improve on the halting pace of the last three decades to make integrated days an available choice for most, rather than the current small percentage, of people with significant disabilities. And, more importantly, these events align with the near unanimous voices of people with disabilities and advocacy organizations. For example, Self Advocates Becoming Empowered has emerged as an influential voice of self-advocates with intellectual disabilities in national policy and funding discussions.

State and National Challenges

Any realist will acknowledge there is potential for hopefulness in government initiatives in the interest of meaningful lives. Realists also know that problems of major proportions exist and are growing in alarming ways. Fiscal crises loom over every idea and sign of progress. Human resource issues are emerging in the American demography unseen in the past. Difficulties in widespread implementation haunt every initiative and have for decades (e.g., Taylor, 1988; Mank, 1994; Wehman et al., 2003). Also, the political landscape changes in unexpected ways. While it is reasonable to be hopeful about some emerging trends in government, it is necessary to be realistic about the problems we face in creating meaningful lives for people with disabilities.

Nationwide, state budget crises imperil the daily implementation of supports that create meaningful daytimes. As tax revenues shrink, governments look for ways to reduce spending, including spending on services for people with disabilities. This creates two problems. First, tight funding restricts access to all services. In some cases, this means people remain on waiting lists and receive no daytime services. In other cases, this means limited choices or a reduction in the services that are received. Tight funding also makes it more difficult for providers of services and government agencies to create and implement improvements for meaningful daytimes that are known to create improvements in quality of life (Braddock et al., 2005). Even as state budgets improve, it may remain difficult to discuss increases in funding and supports in the interest of greater access and implementation of improvements.

Federal budget crises and budget deficits create another obvious problem. While this threatens federally funded services, and general aid to states overall, it particularly can affect Medicaid and Social Security. These are the largest sources of funding for supports for people with disabilities, and as such, entire lives, including daytime supports, may be at risk. Even if they are not at risk, then funding crises pose additional barriers to access and improved quality as it becomes difficult to invest in improvement while services are restricted.

Initiatives that have been created are not trouble free. There is little widespread implementation of individualized budgets and employment initiatives. Initiatives such as transition from school to adult life, supported employment, the Ticket to Work program, and others remain excellent ideas. Yet the pace of implementation lags well behind the known potential for quality outcomes. There are many challenges to implementing these changes (Kiernan, Halliday, & Boeltzig, 2004), and implementation varies significantly from state to state (Liu, Ireys, White, & Black, 2004). For example, ideas that improve employment outcomes, such as customized employment, self-employment, and use of natural supports, are difficult to implement with high staff turnover and limits to available training (Callahan, Shumpert, & Mast, 2002; Griffin & Hammis, 2003).

There are problems in implementing known innovations at the local level. These problems include large agencies operating large facilities and other traditional models of services, still lacking in incentives from state and federal levels to convert to individualized support services (Rogan et al., 2001).

Human resources for employees who support people with disabilities are an emerging problem that will require new thinking. The current problem is already considerable. Direct support professionals (DSPs) are underpaid and not well trained. Due to service funding rates, it has been difficult for organizations that provide services to pay well enough to retain staff and improve the quality of services. This creates an additional problem. Because of high turnover and low wages, it is difficult to keep and train staff in the host of new ideas and service improvements (Wehman et al., 2005). As a result, the human resource that supports people with disabilities is constantly relearning basic support skills rather than fully incorporating innovations into supports for daily life. This human resource problem is widely agreed to become bigger in the future. As baby boomers age, the need for personal supports and services will increase substantially. This will create even greater competition for DSPs in an environment where the positions are not attractive for the long term because of wage issues and limited career advancement.

In combination, these problems—budget crises, implementation difficulties, and human resource issues—pose serious long-term problems for people with disabilities and their families. They combine to threaten basic access to supports, leave individuals and families with limited choices, and impede the implementation of new methodologies. And, these structural problems coexist with the advances toward meaningful lives rooted in government initiatives.

INTRIGUING POSSIBILITIES

This context, given the mix of government activity and pressing, even confounding problems, is further complicated by the quality of innovations and improvements for creating and supporting meaningful days. The past innovations of person-centered planning, transition from school to adult life, and supported employment are being improved upon every year. As such, we find ourselves at a time when innovations are developing at a much faster rate than the quality of implementation. In particular, self-determination, as well as innovations in employment and typical community living, creates intriguing possibilities and promise.

Self-determination has changed, and is changing the landscape for the potential for meaningful daytimes. The idea of people with disabilities being in charge of their own lives should have seemed obvious, but the reality of implementing this idea was very different. Improvements in ways to create and implement person-centered plans continue to evolve. Strategies for creating and making available real choices for people with disabilities allows these individuals to live a more personalized lifestyle. Allowing individuals with disabilities, their families, and their allies to control resources for the individual creates an entirely different relationship between people with disabilities and those paid to support them. That is, people with disabilities become the decision makers about services and quality rather than simple recipients offered by government and provider agencies. The phrase "Nothing about us without us" takes on new meaning with every life changed and every story told.

Twenty years ago, the notion of integrated employment with ongoing supports captured the imagination of a generation of people with disabilities, families, advocates, practitioners, government policy makers, and communities. Today, the notion of integrated and supported employment has been improved upon again and again in meaningful ways. Natural supports in the workplace, employer leadership, self-employment, and customized employment are emerging as creative options. Technology removes barriers to employment and creates possibilities where few existed before. Support strategies continue to evolve, becoming both more personal and less intrusive at the same time. A far greater variety of kinds of work and lifelong learning are becoming possible for people with significant disabilities. Ideas have improved upon ideas that came before, creating newer possibilities. Increasing numbers of agencies are pursuing organizational change with a commitment to push the system, break away from traditional models, and create individualized supports for all, including those with the most severe disabilities.

Universal design in the context of typical community sits on the horizon as another intriguing possibility. When, thanks to ADA, it was finally understood that curb cuts benefited everyone in the community, many people thought they understood the notion of universal design. Yet, examples and innovations are bound to make the point again, calling to ask how the principle applies to all environments, services, and activities. In a way, the idea of universal design is similar to emerging innovations that enhance the capacity of the typical and generic communities and systems, so everyone benefits. Universal design has been first about physical environments and is now expanding to technology. Voice recognition systems, hands-free telephones, personal digital assistants, computerized "smart systems" in vehicles and homes, talking computers, electronic kiosks in airports, global positioning systems, accessibility of the Internet, talking books, digital photography, and wireless networking all extend the very notion of universal design well beyond everyone's early understanding of the value.

At the same time, discussion and development of ways to enhance the capacity of the workplace and every community setting to support, and not just accommodate, people with disabilities with new methods that benefit everyone, continues. What is the capacity of the employer community to support everyone? How can it be enhanced? Perhaps special employment systems for people with disabilities are not needed as much as employment systems that create and support the employment of everyone who wants a job. Many people with disabilities have discovered they do not need or want specialized housing; instead, many individuals want and need housing on one floor, near quality health care, with easy access to the environment, and meaningful and enjoyable activities. Individuals want—and benefit from—employers who support all of their employees with flexible schedules. Jobs that capitalize on each person's talents, provide personalized training based on the way each person learns, offer counseling services, give opportunities for massage therapy at work, are flexible with health care options and with family leave when health care is needed, celebrate the unique contributions of each employee, and accommodate individual differences, are ideal. A special electrical system and power grid for people with disabilities is never needed. What is needed is a power system that works for everyone, including people with disabilities. The emerging possibility now is that all community roles, activities, employment, and community services can be thought of from a universal design standpoint.

RECOMMENDATIONS

This convergence of events, problems, and possibilities may be a cause to be perplexed. Intrigue with the possible service improvements is combined with hope from emerging policy and concern about fiscal and other problems. This combination of possibilities, hope, and concern also creates uncertainty for support personnel in a variety of roles. The responsibilities of case managers, personal assistants, DSPs, school personnel, and other provider personnel are less clear as we seek to implement better ideas for self-determination and improved individual outcomes. There is a need for all involved: providers (e.g., employment, day services, residential, service coordinators), individuals, families, and government personnel to find new ways of collaborating with one another, and new ways of combining resources.

While the problems of underemployment and segregation will require careful attention and new thinking, it is also apparent that self-determination, a wider range of personal choices along with new understanding about community and supports, provide a clear sense of mission. The path for continued improvement in the quality of meaningful daytimes for people with significant disabilities will require relentless movement toward the initiatives described below.

There remains significant work to confront the challenges that remain to creating employment and meaningful daytimes for adults with severe disabilities. There is need for implementation of existing policies and creation of new policies, in order to promote integrated options, consumer control, and meaningful lives. There is need for increased flexibility of funding streams, and the need to create policies and practices that direct resources and energy away from segregated options and toward inclusive ones. As part of this effort, there is need to incorporate increased consumer control and choice.

At the state and local levels, it is important to identify best practices and strategies for overcoming barriers and to disseminate information about these barriers, so that states and local agencies can learn from each other.

Specifically, the following recommendations are offered for greater progress toward meaningful lives.

1. *Align funding priorities with existing and emerging policy.* State and federal policy and government initiatives emphasize integration and productivity. Aligning funding to support these outcomes is needed. In residential services, funding of institutions and large congregate settings has given way to more personalized living settings. The same trend is needed in daytime and employment services.

2. *Invest in innovations.* Customized employment, self-employment, personalized budgets, and related ideas have proven their value for small numbers of people with disabilities. Focused investment in these innovations, in order to improve the quality of personal outcomes as well as create access to integrated outcomes, is needed for greater numbers of people with disabilities.

3. *Invest in self-advocacy.* The voice of self-advocacy in state and national policy is emerging. It will be important for state and federal government to invest in supporting the participation and leadership of people with disabilities in policy and implementation decisions.

4. *Invest in transition from school to employment and integrated lifestyles.* Increasingly, schools are emphasizing successful transition from school to

adult life. If schools emphasize inclusive outcomes, then segregated settings are less needed as a place for people to go during the day. And, employment outcomes begin while people are young and create a basis for a lifetime of working and contributing in the community.

This book has been about the need for and clear possibility of meaningful lives—living, working, learning, and socializing in fully integrated settings. There is clarity in the direction of policy. There is clarity from advocates and self-advocates. It is time to shape the implementation of public policy around this clarity and the voice of people with disabilities in order to create and support meaningful lives.

REFERENCES

Americans with Disabilities Act of 1990, PL 101-336, 42 U.S.C. §§ 12101 *et seq.*

Braddock, D., Hemp, R., & Rizzolo, M.C. (2005). *The state of the states in developmental disabilities 2005.* Boulder, CO: Coleman Institute for Cognitive Disabilities.

Butterworth, J., Fesko, S.L., & Ma, V. (2000). Because it was the right thing to do: Changeover from facility-based services to community employment. *Journal of Vocational Rehabilitation, 14*(1), 23–35.

Callahan, M., Shumpert, N., & Mast, M. (2002). Self-employment, choice and self-determination. *Journal of Vocational Rehabilitation, 17*(2), 75–85.

Dreilinger, D., Gilmore, D.S., & Butterworth, J. (2001). National day and employment service trends in mental retardation/developmental disability agencies. *Research to Practice, 7*(3).

Griffin, C., & Hammis, D. (2003). *Making self-employment work for people with disabilities.* Baltimore: Paul H. Brookes Publishing Co.

Individuals with Disabilities Education Act of 1990, PL 101-476, 20 U.S.C. §§ 1400 *et seq.*

Individuals with Disabilities Education Improvement Act of 2004, PL 108-446, 20 U.S.C. §§ 1400 *et seq.*

Kiernan, W.E., Halliday, J.F., & Boeltzig, H. (2004). *Economic engagement: An avenue to employment for individuals with disabilities.* Boston: University of Massachusetts, Institute for Community Inclusion.

Liu, S., Ireys, H., White, J., & Black, W. (2004). *Enrollment patterns and medical expenditures for Medicaid Buy-In participants in five states.* Washington, DC: Mathematica Policy Research, Inc.

Mank, D.M. (1994). The underachievement of supported employment: A call for reinvestment. *Journal of Disability Policy Studies, 5*(2), 1–24.

Mank, D., Cioffi, A., & Yovanoff, P. (1998). Employment outcomes for people with severe disabilities: Opportunities for improvement. *Mental Retardation, 36*(3), 205–216.

Metzel, D., Butterworth, J., & Gilmore, D.S. (2004). The national survey of community rehabilitation providers, FY2002–2003 Report 3: Involvement of CRPs in the Ticket to Work and the Workforce Investment Act. *Research to Practice, 41,* 1–10.

Migliore, A., Mank, D., Grossi, T., & Rogan, P. (submitted for publication). Integrated employment or sheltered workshops: Preferences of adults with intellectual disabilities, their families, and staff. *Journal of Vocational Rehabilitation.*

Murphy, S.T., Rogan, P.M., Handley, M., Kincaid, C., & Royce-Davis, J. (2002). People's situations and perspectives eight years after workshop conversion. *Mental Retardation, 40*(1), 30–40.

Olmstead v. L.C. and E.W., 98 U.S. 536 (1999).

Pledl, R. (2005). *Schwartz v. Jefferson County.* Paper presented at the Annual Association for Persons in Supported Employment Conference, Mobile, Alabama.

Rehabilitation Act Amendments of 1998, PL 105-220, 29 U.S.C. §§ 701 *et seq.*

Rehabilitation Act of 1973, PL 93-112, 29 U.S.C. §§ 701 *et seq.*

Rizzolo, M.C., Hemp, R., Braddock, D., & Pomeranz-Essley, A. (2004). *The state of the states in developmental disabilities.* Retrieved December 12, 2006, from http://www.ajepartners.com/Braddock%20State%20of%20the%20States%202004.pdf

Rogan, P., Grossi, T., Mank, D., Haynes, D., & Thomas, F. (2001). *Report for the president's task force on the employment of adults with disabilities: A comparison of wages, hours, benefits, and integration between former sheltered workshop participants who are now in supported employment.* Bloomington, IN: Indiana Institute on Disability and Community.

Sowers, J.A., McLean, D., & Owens, C. (2002). Self-directed employment for people with developmental disabilities: Issues, characteristics, and illustrations. *Journal of Disability Policy Studies, 13*(2), 97–104.

Taylor, H. (2000). *Conflicting trends in employment of people with disabilities, 1986–2000.* Retrieved January 5, 2007, from http://www.harrisinteraction.com/harris_poll/index.asp?PID=121

Taylor, S.J. (1988). Caught in the continuum: A critical analysis of the principle of the least restrictive environment. *Journal for the Association for Persons with Severe Handicaps, 13*(1), 41–53.

Ticket to Work and Workforce Incentives Improvement Act of 1999, PL 106-170, 42 U.S.C. §§ 1305 *et seq.*

U. S. Department of Health & Human Services. (2001). *New Freedom Initiative: Fulfilling America's promise to Americans with disabilities.* Retrieved June 4, 2006, from http://www.hhs.gov/newfreedom/

Wehman, P., Mank, D., Rogan, P., Luna, J., Kregel, W., et al. (2005). Employment and productive life roles. In K. C. Lakin & A. Turnbull (Eds.), *National goals and research for people with intellectual and developmental disabilities* (pp. 149–178). Washington, DC: American Association on Mental Retardation.

Wehman, P., Revell, G., & Brooke, V. (2003). Competitive employment: Has it become the "first choice" yet? *Journal of Disability Policy Studies, 14*(3), 163–173.

Index

Page references to figures and tables are indicated by *f* and *t*, respectively.